I Wasn't Strong Like This When I Started Out

TRUE STORIES OF
BECOMING
A NURSE

Edited by
LEE GUTKIND

Foreword by
KAREN WOLK FEINSTEIN

InFACT | BOOKS
Pittsburgh

Requests for permission to reproduce material
from this work should be sent to:
  Rights and Permissions
  In Fact Books
  C/O Creative Nonfiction Foundation
  5501 Walnut Street, Suite 202
  Pittsburgh, PA 15232

Cover design by Tristen Knight
Text design by Heidi Whitcomb

ISBN: 978-1-937163-12-9

Printed in the United States of America

CONTENTS

ACKNOWLEDGMENTS

I *Wasn't Strong Like This When I Started Out* is the third in a series of narrative books on science and medicine supported by the Jewish Healthcare Foundation, whose primary mission is to support healthcare services, education, and research and to encourage medical advancement and protect vulnerable populations. On behalf of the Creative Nonfiction Foundation and the contributors to this collection, I would like to thank Karen Wolk Feinstein and her colleagues at the Jewish Healthcare Foundation—particularly Nancy Zionts and Carla Barricella—not only for their ongoing encouragement and support but also for their faith in the power of true stories and bold voices.

Any book is the work of many people. I would like to thank, most of all, Chad Vogler for his editorial skill and extraordinary dedication to the project; Hattie Fletcher for her advice and counsel; Anjali Sachdeva and Em Maier for their editorial assistance; Donna Brown Hogarty for fact checking; Melissa Irr Harkes for her legal counsel; and the entire staff at In Fact Books. In addition, I am grateful to the Juliet Lea Hillman Simonds Foundation; the Consortium for Science, Policy, and Outcomes and the Hugh Downs School of Human Communication at Arizona State University; and the Pennsylvania Council on the Arts, all of whose ongoing support has been essential to the Creative Nonfiction Foundation's success.

Some names and identifying details have been changed to protect the identities of people and institutions mentioned in these essays.

INTRODUCTION:
The Anonymous, Irreplaceable Nurse

Lee Gutkind

I have written five books about the medical world over the past two decades, and for each book I have plunged myself into the medical center milieu, living the life about which I was writing—psychiatry, pediatrics, surgery, genetics—from varied points of view. And yet, as I sat down to write this introduction, it was difficult to remember many of the nurses in those stories. Doctors and patients—yes. But the nurses are somehow and for some reason not nearly as clear in my memory.

And another thing—over the past few months, I have been back in the hospital for personal reasons: my mother, ninety-three, was admitted because of suspected heart problems; my son, twenty-one, experienced severe intestinal problems and was admitted; my uncle, eighty-six, and one of my oldest friends, Frank, seventy-two, were dying. Sitting and visiting with these four people who had been in my life for nearly as long as I could remember, I saw very few doctors, but I remember quite vividly who they were and what we talked about. Doctors are deity. They're the guys who count—so we have been led to believe.

Yet they could not function in most venues without nurses. And where in my recollections are the helpful and caring nurses who were constantly in and out of the rooms, changing bandages, arranging schedules for testing, giving and explaining medications, calming the anxieties of patient and family? I cannot tell you what any of these nurses looked like, what their names were, where they came from. All I remember, and all that mattered, is that my loved ones were tended to by these irreplaceable yet (at least to me) semi-invisible people. I felt comforted and secure because they were there, yet took them for granted.

That these professionals are so unnoticed is a significant aspect of nursing that both intrigues and troubles me. There are over 2.7 million working registered nurses (RNs) in the United States—not to mention our many licensed practical nurses (LPNs) and licensed vocational nurses (LVNs)—compared with about 690,000 physicians and surgeons. There are more nurses in the United States than engineers (over 2 million) or accountants and auditors (1.2 million). Think of it: more than half of 1 percent of the entire US population are nurses—and the number of nurses is expected to grow over the next half-dozen years to nearly 3.5 million, due in part to the more than 75 million baby boomers who increasingly require residential, home, hospital, or hospice care. Why do we take their work for granted? Surely everyone shall realize that nurses are the indispensible and anchoring element in our healthcare system.

Of course, we all know nurses; I mean, we know them as people. They work out at the gyms we go to, live in the apartment across the hall or in the house around the corner, hang out at the local Starbucks, take courses at the nearby universities where they work on advanced degrees; they are everywhere, men and women of all ages, from twenty-one-year-old graduates to middle-aged folks returning to the workforce or starting new professions. Nurses are ubiquitous in society. We know that they help us, and we know that they are often the key forces who keep our loved ones (and us!) alive. And yet, we know very little about them—professionally.

There are many reasons for this lack of awareness, foremost of which might be the fact that nurses no longer wear distinctive uniforms, so we don't readily notice or remember them. No more white hats with the red crosses or white nursing oxfords. Running shoes, clogs, and blue scrubs, sometimes with lab coats, pretty much constitute the wardrobe of all medical personnel in the hospital, nurses included. And the larger the medical center, the more categorized and confined the nurses become. While doctors, administrators, social workers, genetic counselors, and others float through the hospital, nurses remain more or less in their assigned, self-contained units. And because the workload is often overwhelming, they rarely leave the floor—or the operating room. Scrub nurses remain in the OR throughout their entire shifts, wearing masks. At one point in time, hospital cafeterias were maintained to serve the medical staff, but now they mostly service the families of patients. Most nurses in medical center settings have little time to sit down and eat meals like "normal" people.

There are also nurses in street clothes—home care nurses, mostly, who tend to the chronically ill or the dying. Nurses often specialize, these days. There are transport nurses assigned to ambulances or helicopters, for example, and transplant or procurement coordinator nurses, not to mention nurse practitioners who fulfill roles once played by physicians. In this collection of essays, you will become intimately involved with many different kinds of nurses from diverse walks of life, nurses of various ages and differing attitudes about their profession. Most of these essays were submitted over a period of a few months in response to a call for manuscripts. We received about two hundred, and most of them were quite excellent. Few nurses receive training in creative writing, and yet the power of the narratives and the clarity of the prose were quite astounding. Perhaps it is because nurses have such compelling stories to tell—and also because the stories they are telling have brewed inside of them for many years (in some cases, decades)—that the stories burst forth with vividness and passion.

But allow me to revisit the idea of and the reasons for nurses' anonymity in some quarters. Nurses tend to keep their experiences to themselves, though they do trust, confide in, and confess to other nurses. I am not saying that there's no friction or animosity among nurses in the workplace. To the contrary, nurses are more critical of one another than are members of any other group in the medical center, including physicians. Nurses have a lot to prove to themselves and others precisely because their work is often not spotlighted. But as hard as they can be on one another, nurses faithfully and forcefully support each other in times of stress, emotion, and need—most especially the veteran nurses who reach out on a regular basis to those who are just entering the profession. This mentoring aspect fades as the nurses mature and fashion their own distinct ways of dealing with difficulty, but there seems to be an affinity and connection between the veterans and the rookies—the head nurses and the newbies.

A head nurse must be the strongest person in the unit, for he or she serves as a role model; at the same time, this person must exhibit tenderness and be attentive to younger nurses, usually recent graduates, especially those who are experiencing a patient's death for the first time. Losing a patient is an initiation, a passage through which all nurses who work in tense and highly demanding environments must travel—a sad and unavoidable voyage that remains forever in the nurse's consciousness.

I observed this passage quite vividly, once, learning from the points of view of both the veteran and the new nurse at a children's hospital I was writing about. A head nurse in the neonatal intensive care unit (NICU) told me this story: a baby died while a brand-new nurse, fresh out of school, twenty-one years old, was caring for him. "I went to be with her right away, even before the baby was dead but when it was clear that death was imminent," the head nurse told me. "I knew that the baby was taken care of. We had other nurses covering that baby at that time, and the social worker was with the mom and dad. So I went to be with that young nurse, who probably needed me more than anybody else did. I asked her, 'Do you want to continue taking care of this baby, or would you like to change assignments?'

"And she didn't say anything, and then I said, 'I really think it would be better for you if you took care of this baby.' She needed to know in the days to come she could go through this whole process. And she did. She was in tears, but she returned to the bedside and picked up the baby and held him. And after the baby died, she picked him up again and held him close to her. She held the baby because Mom and Dad could not hold the baby. Mom wanted to remember the baby the way he was when he was not sick. So she helped the family by doing that. But she also helped herself, because she was able to go through the whole process with this little baby and family. And after the baby died, she carried him downstairs to the morgue, where he was going to have his autopsy.

"She went through all of the sequences. And I think that the right decision was made for her to continue with that baby, but for her also to take note—to know that she had someone to talk to. Because you need to know that you are not going through this alone. That's too hard. You see, this has happened to me. I have been that nurse taking care of the baby, and the baby has died, and I learned that the best thing was to do all you could for the baby and for the family, extend yourself to the maximum—because in the end you have to live with yourself."

Weeks later, I met the nurse whose story the head nurse had told. "It was the first time I had ever dealt with anybody professionally or personally who was dying," she told me. "But that day they assigned me to take care of Adam. About two hours after I started, they did his EEG (elecroencephalogram), and everything was flat and nonreactive, and the parents decided that they were going to withdraw support. Right then and there, I just got a knot in my stomach because I knew that this was my first time. *Don't cry; don't do anything*—it was like I was really trying to talk myself into holding back from feeling anything. And then the parents didn't want to hold him, and as bad as I felt and as teary eyed as I was, I decided I wanted to hold him; somebody had to hold him. I just felt it was unfair to allow him to die alone.

"Since then, I have gone through this experience two or three more times. And it gets easier—not so much easier emotionally, but you are in better control of it. You might only cry one or two tears instead of bawling your eyes out. It is not as gut wrenching as it is the first time. It never feels better—it is just easier to hold back until you are driving home by yourself and nobody can see you crying."

As I thought back to that conversation with the young nurse, I realized that the nurses in this collection are telling very similar stories. They are stories about nursing, of course, but also stories about aloneness and strength. These essays are survivor stories, narratives about how to get through the trauma and drama and the awful sadness that come from the day-to-day work in their profession. And I should add that nurses usually don't share their stories with the outside world because they want to spare friends and family the sadness and shock they are forced to endure as parts of their jobs. More than anything, they want to leave the pressure and the scars of their profession behind them when they leave work at the end of a shift.

As I have said, nurses have been anonymous to many people—and for understandable reasons. But in this collection of essays, they are sharing their secret up-and-down lives with the world. Each essay tells a different story, but all of the essays have a common theme: no matter how difficult nurses' lives or how secret their suffering, becoming a nurse entails movement into another dimension of strength and character and persistence; it is a path of irreplaceable and often unacknowledged service to society and humanity.

All nurses will understand the message inherent in the title of this book. It is the theme of survival, the theme of maturity, the theme of selflessly treating and healing all patients in any way possible, whether the credit that is due is forthcoming or not. No matter what your age, race, or sexual orientation is, you become a different, stronger, and more capable and well-adjusted person than you ever imagined possible, once you become a nurse. You have reached a plateau of service and empathy heretofore unimaginable. As Tilda Shalof expressed in her essay, "I See You," all nurses say with confidence and know for certain that this phrase is true: "I wasn't strong like this when I started out."

FOREWORD:
The Art of Meeting Patient Need

Karen Wolk Feinstein

Nurses devoted to good patient care regularly encounter systems that fail them and their patients. Two singular incidents have revealed to me the sometimes desperate lives of nurses. I think of the nurse, for example, who could no longer endure the frequency with which the pharmacy either overlooked or inaccurately filled medications. She demonstrated her work-around to me, reaching up through a tile in the dropped ceiling to expose a comprehensive cache of drugs—drugs she had retrieved when patients were discharged before their meds could be dispensed. Another nurse, frustrated in her attempts to halt the use of a new and cheaper surgical tape, the adhesive of which left patients with quarter-size blisters, called the pharmaceutical company herself and received verification of their quality problems. She alerted a board member and saved many patients from infection and discomfort.

Nurses like these have honed the art of meeting patient need while dealing with their own emotional issues in this challenging profession. In almost any job, there are moments of great personal satisfaction and positive excitement, as well as moments of the reverse. And there are many mundane tasks in between. But for nurses, the ability to extract meaning from the good, the bad, the disappointing, and the boring adds a dimension that sets their work apart.

The nurses whose stories appear in this collection display an extraordinary ability to extract that meaning from participation in a new birth; from helping patients to cope with pain, disfigurement, and disability; or from easing the passage at the end of life. Their stories provide us with insight into the ways the nurses themselves are changed by their daily intimacy with life, death, and suffering.

These stories also highlight the complicated role that nurses play in the hierarchy of medical treatment, where their insight and knowledge about the patient can be circumvented by less engaged physicians and administrators. As authors, the nurses can say what they cannot voice in the cultures of their hospitals and practices. Equally, the stories have meaning on many levels: ethical, cultural, spiritual, managerial, and practical; they have educational implications for all members of the medical team, and they promote inter-professional understanding.

The stories also remind us that our nurses share in our medical dramas; patients may have starring but not central roles. In my own and in my family members' hospitalizations, nurses made the major contributions to our healing. They can buffer or exacerbate the helplessness and dependency of the sick. Nurses play key roles in all healthcare settings: from primary care practice to specialty and emergency care to rehab, long-term care, and hospice. Good healthcare is built on good nursing.

At the Jewish Healthcare Foundation and our operating arms—the Pittsburgh Regional Health Initiative and Health Careers Futures—we are pleased to offer a number of Champions programs for nurses who wish to become leaders in the effort to improve the quality, safety, and efficiency of care in their settings. These nurses learn key quality-improvement techniques and apply them in major projects, which are captured and recorded in one of our publications or two-minute Teachable Moment videos. All are available on our website, www.prhi.org. We are continually awed by the achievements of these nurse Champions.

The nursing profession deserves a volume devoted to it. It is our pleasure to work again with Creative Nonfiction and to bring to you this volume of up-close and personal stories of the wonder that is the life of a nurse.

KAREN WOLK FEINSTEIN, *PhD, is president and CEO of the Jewish Healthcare Foundation and the Pittsburgh Regional Health Initiative. She is editor of the recent book* Moving Beyond Repair: Perfecting Healthcare.

HITTING THE BONE

Eddie Lueken

Giving a patient a shot for the first time is a right of passage. A nursing student's opportunity finally comes, but she finds the task more challenging than she imagined it would be.

Mabel Tate looked dead. As a nursing student, my assessment skills were admittedly limited, but the comatose Miss Tate looked considerably worse than the only dead person I had seen in my nineteen years. That person was my fifty-year-old grandfather, who was gregariously alive one day and embalmed the next. Laid out in his dark blue suit in a mahogany, satin-lined casket, he wore such a pleasant expression that it seemed he had enjoyed his massive heart attack. Miss Tate's face expressed no enjoyment—a justified demeanor, it seemed, when I considered her situation.

I reviewed my homework notes, written on a pocket-sized file card: "Patient diagnosis: Breast cancer with bony mets. Mets is short for metastasis and that means the spread of cancer from one part of the body to another. The primary cancer started in her breast and then spread to her bones." For the next three days I would be taking care of Miss Tate from eight in the morning until noon. A staff nurse and my clinical instructor, Ms. Wilson, were ultimately responsible for Miss Tate's care, even though I would do all the work while they darted in and out of the room, ensuring I did no harm. We had just moved on from the fundamentals of nursing—bed making, bed baths, how to turn patients like they were logs—to giving injections and inserting urinary catheters. Because my patient already had a catheter and was on no routine medications, this assignment was bad news for me. Another day of basics. When would I get to start an IV? Give a shot? Milk someone's chest tube? So far, nursing school had been a boring, bloodless disappointment. I was tired of memorizing the names of nerves, muscles, and bones. I was ready to do something dramatically heroic.

I didn't know what cancer looked like or how it killed a person, and I wasn't interested in learning. Of course, I was aware it could be lethal, but I did not understand that advanced malignant tumors grow wildly, sucking nourishment out of tissues and bones, shutting down vital organs, and generally starving their hosts, like Miss Tate, to death. But even aggressive cancers seemed to wage war in slow motion when compared to a hemorrhaging trauma victim, who could be saved only by decisive, cool-headed people willing to get blood under their fingernails. Curing someone with cancer required patience and the analytical skills of a champion chess player—not as thrilling as defibrillating an arrested heart into beating again. I had enrolled in nursing school to get in on the action. Denture care for someone who was lying in the fetal position, looking as though she'd never eat again, wasn't the kind of action I had in mind.

The off-going night nurse informed me that the physician had written a DNR order on Miss Tate. When I looked confused, she said, "That means do not resuscitate. She's a no-code." Calling a code mobilized a team of people who sprinted from the emergency room or the ICU, arriving at the patient's bedside out of breath and ready to jumpstart a heart or inflate a pair of lungs. Full of adrenaline, they shoved everything from their path with such force that bedside commodes and tables whirl-blasted out of the room. The team members felt duped when they were met at the patient's door and told, "Never mind, she's a no-code"; after all, they were important people who saved lives better than the rest of us. They would yell at the floor staff and report the false alarm to the house supervisor, who would yell at the staff again. To avoid all the yelling, staff posted reminders like the one over Miss Tate's bed that read, in bold, red letters, DNR. In other words, don't bother. My patient didn't need a code team; she needed an undertaker.

While it was true that I didn't even know how to initiate a code blue, how was I supposed to learn with DNR patients? Was there a shortage of sick people who needed to be resuscitated? I was paying the college to teach me how to keep people alive; I already possessed the skills to let someone die. I earned tuition money by bussing tables at a steak house and came home smelling like greasy T-bones and A.1. sauce, odors that the hottest, soapiest shower couldn't eliminate. I didn't spend my evenings wearing a cowboy hat and getting screamed at by the restaurant's hostile dishwasher (he hated the way I stacked plates) so I could learn how to disimpact a sluggish bowel or measure the diameter of a bedsore.

I leaned in for a closer look at her face and, in case she could hear, introduced myself. "Miss Tate, I'm Eddie, a nursing student, and I'll be taking care of you today." Nothing in her stony, pale face indicated the slightest response. I'd seen more lifelike faces at a wax museum. Someone had braided her silver, waist-length hair into a ponytail that hung off the side of the bed. Eyes closed, she wore a disapproving grimace, which I took personally. Maybe she was disgusted by what she heard going on around her. Nurses said just about anything in the presence of unconscious patients, and perhaps Miss Tate had become unwillingly privy to someone's yeast infection or extramarital affair.

As I pulled back the sheets, I thought that rigor mortis had already set in; or had she begun to decompose? No, I was pretty sure that decomposition could occur only in genuinely dead bodies, but I'd have to look up rigor mortis when I got home. What else could have accounted for her contracted legs and arms? I thought a bed bath would be impossible; hosing her off might work better.

Spidery blue veins ran across the milky, transparent skin of her eighty-pound body like a thousand little tributaries joining a river. To touch her was startling. A damp hospital gown clung to her cold, wet skin. I assumed that the black bruises in the inner aspects of both elbows were due to repeated needle sticks for lab work. What a pity to poke her every day. Did Miss Tate's doctor think it was a good idea to discontinue lifesaving measures but not her lab work?

It occurred to me that she may very well have stopped breathing while I was fumbling around with my file cards, she was so still. I imagined my instructor walking in to find me trimming the toenails of a dead woman. She would say: "Miss Lueken, would you step out into the hall, please?" where she would explain that my patient had died without my noticing and suggest that I consider a career in retail or look into promotion opportunities at the steak house.

I leaned in closer, positioning my ear beneath Miss Tate's nose, watching and waiting for her rigid chest to move up and down. I deduced that she was breathing; barely, but she was definitely breathing. Her respirations were six per minute, pretty low for a normal person. I didn't know if that was normal for a dying person. Just taking her vital signs was an ordeal. Although I had repeatedly inflated the blood pressure cuff, I heard nothing. Pumping up the cuff and squeezing her twig of an arm, then prying open her bent elbow to place my stethoscope on her brachial pulse, I wondered if I might fracture a bone.

"Miss Lueken, how's it going in here?" Known for her no-nonsense demeanor, Ms. Wilson was uncommonly lean and fit. She was not as intimidating as Mrs. Shuman (a retired army nurse who had already kicked five students out of the program), but Ms. Wilson wasn't the nurturing type, either.

"I'm not sure how to help this woman," I said, shrugging.

"Let's see your care plan," she said, referring to a document dreaded by all nursing students. Every Monday, a student received her patient assignment for the week, along with enough information—such as diagnosis and daily treatments—to formulate a comprehensive plan for the patient's care. This step-by-step approach listed a patient's problems in the first column, identified corresponding treatments or nursing actions in the second, and described an evaluation of each action in the third. We dreaded the care plan because, as we saw it, our patients didn't have enough problems for us to write out lengthy, impressive-looking plans. It was tempting to fabricate a few problems, but when a professor suspected creative or fictitious writing, the student received a failing grade. Getting a zero on a care plan was the kiss of death in nursing school, as the only way to bring up one's average was to make all As on the subsequent care plans—something unheard of.

A well-written nursing care plan defied common sense. Only someone with no self-esteem or a low IQ filled in the blank columns properly. Unlike physicians, who were qualified to diagnose, nurses were forced to use such submissive language that a care plan read like an apology for even having noticed that something was wrong with a patient. According to the rules of care plan writing, the author should replace all strong verbs with "appears." A patient could be found in his bed, recently decapitated, and the care plan would read: "Problem: Pt's body appears to have been separated from pt's head as evidenced by gap between the body and head. Scarlet fluid noted running down neck area and staining pillowcase."

The care plan authorities allowed us to use direct quotes from patients, however, to support our unreliable observations. Perhaps I could have been trusted to accurately describe Miss Tate's expression in order to list her primary problem, such as: "Patient appears unhappy about her terminal condition, as evidenced by fixed facial grimace." If I could have gotten a direct quote out of Miss Tate, I think she would have said something like, "Leave me alone." That kind of feedback could be listed as another problem: "Appears depressed about her terminal condition." Now that I was sure she wasn't dead, I needed to come up with a problem that submissively stated, somehow, that she looked really bad. I had considered writing: "Appears to be suffering from premature rigor mortis" as a problem, but hesitated until I could get to a medical dictionary to ascertain whether such a term existed.

As it was, my care plan listed one problem: "Appears unstable as evidenced by abnormal vital signs." The action column had one entry that stated my intention to monitor her vital signs closely. I handed the mostly blank, crumpled paper to Ms. Wilson.

"Is this what you plan to do all day for your patient? Take her vital signs every two hours?" Ms. Wilson asked.

What else could a person do for Miss Tate? She wasn't hungry, she didn't need assistance to take a walk, she didn't need education about her disease. Although she was dying, she didn't vent about her anger or depression, a dynamic we were taught to expect from coherent terminally ill people.

"Huh, I don't know what else to do, other than bathe her and change her sheets."

"Did you read about bone cancer?"

"Yes," I said.

"Tell me what you know about bone cancer, then."

"That it's a common site for cancer to spread to. It may cause fractures and sometimes chemotherapy can stop the growth," I recited from my file card.

"Anything else?"

I was out of answers.

"Bone cancer is painful, Miss Lueken. Do you think your patient might be in pain?" Ms. Wilson asked.

"I don't know. How could I tell?"

"Look at the whole picture and use your head. Her cancer is so far advanced that she's a DNR. Her facial expression is not a content or peaceful one. When in doubt, err on the side of assuming that someone in her condition needs pain meds. She has morphine ordered every four hours, and she's overdue because the night nurse refused to give her last injection." Ms. Wilson lectured me over the patient's head while leaning against a bedrail. Was it my imagination, or did Miss Tate just nod her head?

"Why?" I asked.

"Narcotics decrease respirations. Because her respirations are already so low, a dose of morphine could hasten her death. What are her respirations now?"

"Six," I said, relieved that I had at least taken her vital signs.

"Anything under nine or ten is considered risky. So what's your call, Miss Lueken?" Crossing her arms, she looked me in the eye. "Should you give a dying woman with advanced bone cancer her pain medication, or withhold it because she may stop breathing?"

My heart raced. I could be giving my first shot! I'd recently cared for a man recovering from a hemorrhoidectomy and a woman who had bunions removed from both feet—two very painful procedures. I had tried to persuade them to take pain shots, but they opted for pills. I needed to give an injection to someone other than Gertrude, the lab dummy.

"You mean we get to decide without calling the doctor?" I asked.

"Yes, it's called a nursing judgment."

I looked at Miss Tate. Did I want to give a shot bad enough to push her over the edge?

"I'll give it," I said, giddy with anticipation.

"Good," Ms. Wilson nodded.

By the time my instructor and I walked to the medication room, the news of my good fortune had spread throughout the floor. Several wide-eyed students peered through the door as Ms. Wilson unlocked the stainless-steel narcotic chest where hundreds of glistening glass vials were lined up in alphabetical order. For two months I had rehearsed for this moment. I unpeeled the syringe package, injected air into the vial, and withdrew 1 cc of morphine. The inch-and-a-half needle seemed about a foot long.

I proudly paraded down the hall, carrying a small metal tray with the syringe of morphine and three alcohol pads. Back at Miss Tate's bedside, I took her respirations once more. They hadn't improved. After turning my patient on her side, I pointed out the bony landmarks and drew an imaginary line on her hip to demonstrate for Ms. Wilson where I planned on giving this shot. She nodded and said, "I'll warn you, as thin as she is, you may hit her bone with the tip of the needle. If that happens, back out a little bit, and then go ahead and inject the medication."

We had learned about hitting the bone during our lecture on injections, but I was good with my hands and imagined that only the brainy, clinically inept students committed that error. Looking at her hip, I knew exactly where to give this shot. I wiped her skin with alcohol in a circular motion, removed the needle cap, and plunged the gleaming needle into the hip of Miss Tate. My wrist bent as though I'd thrown a dart at a bull's-eye. The needle penetrated her skin and glided through her muscle. It was easy— that is, until I felt the abrupt vibration of the needle running headlong into the old woman's hip bone.

It stopped hard and fast, akin to a car hitting a concrete wall. My stomach lurched. Mabel Tate's dreadful predicament—her unrelenting pain, her reliance on strangers, her debilitating condition that had stolen her voice— all of it was buried in that brittle, cancerous bone; the bone I had jabbed with the beveled edge of a big needle. All of it reverberated through my hand.

My hand froze, and my face went hot. So confident that I wouldn't hit the bone, I hadn't bothered to pay attention to Ms. Wilson's instructions. "Huh, it feels like I hit her bone."

"Just back the needle out a little," she said. I considered leaving the needle sticking out of Miss Tate's hip and moving aside for Ms. Wilson to take over. I didn't want to do this pitiful woman any more harm. I hoped that if I hesitated long enough, Ms. Wilson would intervene.

"Eddie, back the needle out and give her the morphine. You know how to do this." The woman overestimated my abilities. I gritted my teeth, pulled the needle back about a quarter of an inch, and pushed the plunger. I couldn't imagine that I deposited the morphine anywhere near where it should be going. After I withdrew the needle, my hands shook so hard that I nearly stuck myself when I tried to recap the now-contaminated needle. Ms. Wilson patted me on the shoulder. "You did fine," she lied.

Afterward, I watched Miss Tate's face, searching for some sign that the pain relief from the morphine had been worth the assault, wondering if my first shot would be her last. Her expression offered no forgiveness. I bathed her, turned her, changed her linens, scrubbed her dentures, and rearranged the pink plastic emesis basin and water pitcher on her over-bed table.

I sat at Miss Tate's bedside, writing a care plan while her respirations slowed in the chilly room without family or other visitors. Worried that my clinical evaluation would reflect my botched attempt at giving an injection, I imagined Ms. Wilson writing something like, "It's too bad that this student had to hurt a dying patient before she could understand the needs of a dying patient." Ms. Wilson, however, would overlook the bone-hitting incident and give me an A on my care plan, which highlighted a problem that I called: "Patient appears to be in pain and generally uncomfortable." I found her comments written in her usual, neat penmanship on the back page: "Eddie, this is a thoughtful assessment designed for the pain management needs of a dying patient. Good job."

Miss Tate died a few hours after I left that day. "She went quietly," the charge nurse told me the next morning, as if my comatose patient had the capacity to become loud and rambunctious at the end.

"Did her expression ever relax? You know, did she look more at peace when she died?" I asked, hoping to assuage my guilt about the painful injection.

"I didn't notice," the nurse said, shaking her head.

On my way down the hall to assess my new patient, I stopped in the room where I'd given my first shot. Someone had turned down the fresh, white cotton bedspread on Mabel Tate's vacated bed in preparation for a new admission. As I stood in the quiet room, it suddenly occurred to me that I might not turn out to be a good nurse. I tried to shake the bad feeling by picturing myself valiantly performing CPR on a trauma victim in the ER, but all I could see was Miss Tate's frown, her spiky shoulders, her long silver hair that someone else had braided for the last time.

A nurse for thirty years, **EDDIE LUEKEN** *received an MFA in creative writing from Spalding University. Her essays have appeared in* The Louisville Review *and the anthology* 21 Peaceful Nurses.

THE HAUNTING

Thomas Schwarz

Following a tragic car accident, an emergency room nurse struggles to overcome posttraumatic stress disorder. When he takes a job in hospice, however, he finds his experience helps him identify with his patients and their loved ones.

Thirty-three years ago, on a lazy summer evening in an emergency room in the suburbs of New York, I chose my first dying patient. An older, more experienced nurse was instructing me in the art and science of triage; her hours of patient explanations and unfailingly accurate assessments could be boiled down to a simple dictum: the worst goes first. The tricky part was to determine within a few seconds, a minute at most, who was at death's door and who was merely impatient and whining the loudest. When it came time to step up and choose my first patient, I guessed right. Or maybe wrong. I'm still not sure.

Two patients had arrived simultaneously. My mentor deferred to me, and I chose the obese, late-middle-aged, wheelchair-bound patient because his complaint seemed benign. He'd told the admission clerk that he'd had a sore throat for several days. In fact, he had the perfect storm of alcoholism and long-term aspirin use for rheumatoid arthritis, the consequences of which were the bulging esophageal varices that tickled his throat like angry, red balloons, growing more taut with each heartbeat of unclotted blood. I didn't foresee that he would die momentarily. As I weaved his wheelchair through the corridor, cluttered with empty stretchers and portable X-ray machines, I asked about his pain. Or perhaps I asked his name, or how long he'd had the sore throat; it was many, many shifts ago, and I can't remember. But I remember the next moment clearly: he lifted his left hand to his throat, coughed deeply once, and turned in his seat to stare into my eyes as he vomited a wave of blood. It didn't have the "coffee grounds" appearance that indicates that the blood has been partially digested in the patient's stomach. No, this bucket of blood—*frank red blood* is the accepted clinical description—came straight up and out of the hemorrhaging varices in explosive gushes that filled his lap and covered his crippled legs. He didn't speak a word. I was too shocked to call for help, not that any drug or procedure could have saved him. He held my eyes with his own, too surprised to be scared, as his barrel chest shuddered with each heave. His hands gripped the wheelchair arms as if he were trying to save himself from slipping away. Moments later, his eyelids relaxed, and an unexpected calmness overtook him. He slipped down in his seat, looking as if nothing in the world could bother him, as if everything would be all right. At last, everything was suddenly fine.

I was not fine. I'm sure I looked gray and shaky as I washed down the wheelchair, pushed the discretely draped patient to the morgue, and completed the paperwork. My ER nursing mentor and the ER physician reassured me, later, that nothing could have quelled his lethal cough or staunched its horrific consequences, but nothing they said could salve my fear that I had missed something. We were there to save lives, not to watch them slip through our fingers, right? Nonetheless, I told them I was OK. After we cleaned up the mess (we never knew the patient's name—he was simply called The Mess), everyone went back to work as if nothing unusual had happened. I didn't understand, at the time, that I wasn't OK. I'd begun the shift with a nursing diploma and a bucket of bravado that someone had kicked over. I'd helplessly watched a life end from an arm's length away. That was the beginning of a long line of endings. After our shift ended, the other nurses collegially took me to the Parkside Tavern and got me numbingly drunk. The next evening, it was business as usual for everyone—except me.

I was barely thirty years old. My parents were alive and well, and even my octogenarian grandparents were still around. I'd never seen someone die until that night. That patient was and to this day remains *my patient*, someone who played out his last few minutes like an actor on my busy ER stage. During my three years at the nursing school from which I'd only recently graduated, the only corpses I saw were on gurneys being wheeled downstairs to the morgue. *Dead*, *dying*, and *death* were words wielded like riding crops by the nursing instructors, who harried the students constantly. A medication error—by far the most prevalent form of medical error, at nine hundred thousand per year—was the easiest way to kill someone, the instructors warned. But I don't recall any instructor who ever admitted that *our* patients might die. They prepared us for hemorrhages, heart attacks, psychiatric emergencies, and birthing catastrophes. We even practiced postmortem care by washing, wrapping, and toe-tagging a latex dummy. But grief, shock, guilt, loss, and uncertainty were not part of the syllabus. We were taught, like the uneasy British during World War II, to keep calm and carry on.

The older nurses, whose refusal to shed tears over appalling events or even to speak of them later, were the models by which I learned to cope with tragedies and incorporate them into my nursing worldview. The nurses seemed, if anything, angry. At what or whom, I hadn't a clue. I didn't want to come off as sensitive, weak, or clueless, so I never spoke of my emotions either. If they were untouched by all the tragedy around us, then by God, I was going to be so-armored, too! I was young and cocky, well trained, and at the top of my ER game. When the screaming started, I would tell myself, *The patients hurt; I don't. Panic is contagious. If I let the patients' feelings become mine, I won't be able to help anyone.* I never let them in. Efficient? Yes. Callow, detached? Maybe. Compassionate? Not yet. It was still a long road to that destination.

In the decades that followed, I honed my emergency skills and clinical knowledge in ERs large and small, urban and rural; I proved my mettle with the "knife and gun club" in the Columbia–Presbyterian Medical Center's emergency department in Manhattan; I learned to save victims of careless hunting accidents and ghastly tractor rollovers. In that adrenaline-fueled atmosphere, patients came and went in a caffeinated blur. There was never enough time to connect in a deep or lasting way. The emergency medical technicians who pushed their stretchers piled with unimaginable tragedy through our doors called their rapid pace scoop and run. In order to keep pace with them, we had our own coping axiom: treat 'em and street 'em.

We sent the more stable patients to the ICU or the general care floors; our primary objective was to not let a patient die.

I distinctly remember the scream of a particularly aggressive doctor. He was directing the care of a dying patient, and his realization of the futility of his team's efforts was mounting. "Not on my time, you bastard—you're not gonna die on me!" he shouted, staring at the cardiac monitor as if he could will its lethal pattern into lifesaving submission. Stunned, I thought this to be a pretty heartless way to treat someone whose life was sloshing in a crimson cascade onto the shoes of the collected trauma specialists who surrounded his stretcher.

I'm not so sure, now, who he was screaming at. His soon-to-be-lifeless patient? The ghosts of past patients who'd slipped from his expert, unrelenting grasp? Maybe a brother who'd been killed at Da Nang or in Detroit while he was still a biology undergrad? Or maybe he was just as scared as I was and, like me, had never spoken a word about his fear to anyone who could help him to sort it out. Maybe his senior resident had exorcised his empathy years ago with the dictum Never let them see you cry.

On a late June evening, seventeen years after I'd started my ER tour of duty, I joined my kids as they chased lightning bugs on our front lawn in rural New York. We shared a second bowl of ice cream after dinner and decided to indulge ourselves by going out to pick up more. For some inexplicable reason, I chose to drive them in our clunky Ford station wagon rather than in my preferred yellow Volkswagen Beetle.

I was turning into our driveway when a drunk and stoned kid on a low-slung, souped-up motorcycle—commonly and appropriately referred to as a crotch rocket—struck my door at more than a hundred miles per hour. We neither saw nor heard his approach, which was odd. Those engines emit a scream that would put a banshee to shame. In the first seconds after his impact, I had no idea why all the windows of my car had blown out. My sole concern was for my kids. "Are you all right?" I shouted. They were miraculously unhurt. Not so, for me. By instinctively bracing myself during the explosive impact, I'd torn several muscles and tendons loose from my right arm and lower left leg. My door wouldn't open, so I slid across the front seat and flopped to the ground. Neither my arm nor leg hurt at that point; they were simply numb and limp.

But I had more on my mind than a diagnosis for this clinical oddity. Somewhere in the warm evening was the person who had watched all his twenty-four years pass before his eyes when his ecstatic speeding was halted by the broad side of my tan, forty-six-hundred-pound Ford LTD station wagon. I searched my garden for the dying motorcycle driver. After what felt like an hour of crawling through weeds, I found him more than fifty feet from the car he'd impaled with his now unrecognizably crumpled motorcycle. His arms and legs lay skewed in a grotesque resemblance to a swastika. I futilely administered my best one-armed CPR as I shouted at him, "You bastard, you're not gonna to die on me! Not in *my* garden!" Years would pass before the irony of this curse would become a moment of enlightenment in my therapeutic journey back to an existence free of pain and posttraumatic stress disorder.

Within a half hour, the local ambulance squad scooped me up and brought me to an ER—fortunately, not to the one where I worked. "What was his name?" I asked repeatedly. The New York state trooper who'd escorted our ambulances repeated the victim's name to me over and over. It wouldn't adhere to my racing brain. Blessedly, some of his words did stick: "It wasn't your fault."

I was undressed, questioned, scanned, X-rayed, and falsely reassured in the ER: "You're OK except for some soft tissue injuries." Nothing could have been further from the truth. Within hours, my shoulder froze; it would stay that way for more than a year. The muscles, tendons, and ligaments in my lower left leg had sustained innumerable microtears when I'd kicked the brake pedal into the firewall. I could wiggle my toes and walk gingerly, and the bones appeared whole on the X-rays. Hence the flippant diagnosis of soft tissue injuries. More important, the nerves from my knee to my toes were numb. My leg had mysteriously gone to sleep. When it began to wake up, a week later, I felt that burning, throbbing, exquisitely painful feeling that occurs when one's circulation returns a few minutes after its deprivation.

The agonizing sensation lasted for the entire summer, robbing me of rest; my usual resilience and sense of humor were displaced by an angry, exhausted zombie nurse. Dozens of hours of agonizing physical therapy later, I could walk without pain and raise my right arm nearly as high and straight over my head as my left. Nearly, but not completely. The price was high, but I had unintentionally earned a measure of empathy that would one day make me a better nurse. But there was more to learn. Never again would I impatiently dismiss a patient's complaints by telling him, "it's just a soft tissue injury." I swore I'd throw the word *just* out of my vocabulary. "This injection will *just* feel like a mosquito bite"; "I'm *just* the nurse"; "You *just* have soft tissue injuries."

On the morning after the crash, not twenty-five yards from where it had occurred, I lay in bed, still dressed in the clothes I'd worn the night before. The summer sunrise soon warmed my bedroom until I began to sweat into the rumpled sheets. Limping outside, I looked down my driveway to the spot where my car had sat, wrecked and steaming, before it was towed away. The occasional commuter's car tooted to me as it whizzed past. Friends and neighbors hadn't yet read the *Poughkeepsie Journal*'s terse report of the tragedy.

I noticed a middle-aged man a few yards down the road. He scanned the ground carefully, periodically picking up something from the gravel margin of the narrow country road. He cradled in his hands a small collection of the shattered pieces of plastic, metal, and glass left behind after the motorcycle was carted away on the flatbed truck, along with my car. He introduced himself as the father of the boy who had died. He said he was sorry for what his son had done and that he'd been expecting it, helplessly waiting for this to happen for a long time. He had told his daughter, long ago, "Someday we're going to get a call about your brother." And last evening, he explained, the call came. His voice teetered on the edge of anguish. His eyes were red rimmed and brimming with hot tears that would soon course down his unshaven cheeks. I'd never seen eyes so tired. He hoped that none of us were injured.

"My kids are all right," I responded.

"Good," he said. "That's a relief."

•   •   •

Over the following weeks and months, I came to understand that not all injuries are visible. Nor do all illnesses have scientific, rational roots. Some surround the heart like barbed wire, never admitting peace or happiness, never allowing the release of residual, unspoken, or misplaced guilt. My psychic pain began with simple, reasonable questions. Why hadn't I seen the motorcyclist in the rearview mirror before I turned into the driveway? Why did he choose to pass in front of and not behind me? Why didn't any of us hear his approach? I wouldn't voice those haunting questions to anyone for many months. Nor did I speak of the collision's deafening boom that replayed in my mind again and again. One night, I became stuck while driving around a busy rotary. I couldn't summon the courage to make a simple turnoff through the thin traffic, so I drove around and around, like a lost soul on a merry-go-round of the damned, for ten minutes. My wife sat silently, patiently, by my side until my hands were cold and clammy from tightly gripping the steering wheel. When I finally exited, I was nauseated and humiliated by my panic.

Worse, I began to experience this feeling whenever I learned that an ambulance was bringing a victim of a motor vehicle accident into my ER. I began to ceaselessly hear crash noises, to the exclusion of all other sounds or voices. My ER expertise was erased, my bravado smothered by my pounding heart. I couldn't evade a patient's pain or panic anymore. I now knew those feelings firsthand, and until I acknowledged them without immature judgment or callous dismissal, I couldn't be truly helpful. In the same vein, I wouldn't be free of my fears until I admitted to my therapist, Marion, my haunting uncertainty about the crash; I spent hours sifting through details and tangled emotions like an archeologist of the soul. She called it a tape loop that had to be cut. Or posttraumatic stress disorder, if you like. Unbroken sleep became my measure for success, a cause for celebration even more profound than my graduation from nursing school. I felt as though I were starting over again, a newbie nurse who now knew what he needed to be a really good nurse: empathy.

I'm out of the ER business now. As I like to explain with a smile, I'm not thirty anymore. The ER pace is far too fast, and those exhausting, necessary trauma skills have outpaced my sixty-three-year-old self's endurance. My brain can't process clinical algorithms and medication dosages fast enough anymore. I can't watch patients die, suddenly and awfully, and later worry that my best wasn't good enough.

On April Fool's Day 2007, I began a new job as a hospice nurse. Saving lives is not an option in hospice, although some patients do defer signing a Do Not Resuscitate order, a tacit admission that they are not entirely ready to die. My job is to help patients pass peacefully and comfortably at home, as is their common preference. The upstate New York hospice agency where I am employed has a fairly steady population of approximately 150 patients, with a predictable winter holiday season rise and post–New Year's decrease—terminally ill patients frequently and inexplicably manage to hold on until the holidays have passed.

The majority of the nurses at our agency work the day shift, during which they provide hands-on care to patients, ensure that they have enough antianxiety and pain-relieving drugs to carry them through until the nurse's next visit, and listen to their final desires, hopes, and fears. I am a strictly nocturnal nurse, on the other hand, who works the sixteen hours from dusk until dawn. In effect, I'm the hospice emergency nurse. After the day-shift nurses have tucked in their patients and gone home to their own happy and healthy families, I wait for the calls from patients whose symptoms—pain, nausea, vomiting, and worst of all, terminal restlessness and agitation—have unexpectedly spun out of control. There's no telling when I'll be summoned. Though we'd like to think that there's some degree of predictability to death and dying, there simply isn't.

My calls come when the patient's caregiver, most often a well-intentioned but inexperienced, overwhelmed, and frightened family member, senses the fear of abandonment that the dying patient feels. Panic, as I said before, is the most contagious of all sicknesses. *Where's our nurse?* they cry. *I'm afraid to give him more morphine, his pain is out of control, and he keeps trying to pull off his clothes and climb out of bed! She's plucking at things on her sheets that aren't there. She takes her oxygen off and tries to yank the tubing out of her arm! She's talking to people who aren't here, who died years ago! He's gurgling, and there's white stuff bubbling out of his nose and mouth. What do I do? He stops breathing for minutes at a time. That can't be right. Is that normal? He's burning up. She's ice cold. My brother wants to take him to the emergency room. We can't wake him up! Please come as quickly as you can!*

Finding my patient's home in the pitch black of a 2:00 a.m. visit is never very hard. It's the only house with every light ablaze and more parked cars than driveway space. I walk from my car to the front door with an air of calm and confidence; someone will be anxiously watching for my arrival. The least confident member of the family, who hopes I have some magic in my big, blue, nylon nursing bag, usually greets me. Inside, I kneel by the patient's bedside. At six foot four, I'm at an appropriate height, in that position, to look into his eyes and not down at him from on high. I hold his hand, smile, and tell him, "My name is Thom, and I'm your nurse. I'm going to do my best to help you right now. What's happening?" The patient is often too lost in his pain or anxiety to answer immediately. He needs to resurface from his awful depths. But I can predict one question that patients never ask, one question that families *always* ask, one question that I can't answer with 100 percent certainty: "When?"

Through my own trials, I now understand the ineffable dread, as well as their inescapable sense of responsibility, that evokes that question. So I sit still, calmly look them in the eyes, and tell them with honesty and certainty, "What you're doing is the best and hardest thing you'll ever do. I respect you for that. I can see that you're doing everything you can. You're doing fine."

Hospice and palliative care services have grown exponentially as our elderly population lives longer and patients with terminal illnesses are increasingly reluctant to die in a hospital or skilled nursing facility— the dreaded "nursing home dump" scenario. Specialized training and a growing body of scientific literature ensure that nurses like me are well prepared for the job. Or are we? When I asked a colleague with seventeen years of hospice experience, "How have you stayed with it for so long?" she smiled with gentle understanding at the deeper meaning of my question.

"If you make it past three years, you'll be fine and stay in it forever," she replied. I also heard her unspoken warning: don't feel bad if you want out after they've wrung every tear out of you.

Although I have already endured that existential loss of innocence, the truth about dying is revealed to me over and over again, night after night. More than three decades of watching countless lives slip away at arm's length has blessed me with the realization that you cannot beat death simply by leading a sane and healthy lifestyle. Everyone dies, and it's rarely easy or pretty. Everyone I've ever known, loved, kissed, sat next to on a bus, watched on TV, or hated in the third grade is going to die. Everyone. I am the midwife to the next life for some. And although hospice nurses are very adept at relieving patients' physical and psychic pains, we're rarely 100 percent successful. Someone's going to suffer. I have lost loved ones and many patients. And I, too, have been scared to death about death.

All too often, new graduates stay in nursing because the recession offers little else to support them. The nursing profession has long acknowledged but never overcome its crippling level of burnout. Mandatory overtime still exists. Nursing's self-help tools are pitiful, demeaning, and far from sufficient to help nurses to recognize and conquer the fear, insecurity, and sadness that rob us of rest, happiness at home, and even our initial, quixotic love of nursing. Our beloved profession becomes just a job all too soon. It needn't be so. Nurses needn't leave the profession, resort to unhealthy coping measures, or become the nurse whose care no one wants for his or her loved one. The tricky part is to learn to be compassionate *and* detached in the right ways and at the right moments. I graduated from nursing school many lifetimes ago. Every night I start again.

THOMAS SCHWARZ, RN, *has been published in the* New York Times Magazine, Newsweek, *the* Journal of the American Medical Association, Writer's Digest, *and numerous other outlets. He has worked in hospitals as large as the Johns Hopkins Cancer Hospital and as small as Northern Dutchess Hospital in Rhinebeck, New York. At present, he is finishing a memoir about men who find it difficult to publicly acknowledge the sexual abuse they endured as boys.*

BECOMING
A NURSE

Laura DeVaney

A recent graduate hopes for a job in labor and delivery, but when job opportunities prove scarce, she finds herself in a postoperative unit for cancer patients who have undergone radical surgeries. But ultimately, she reflects, nursing is nursing: "Life is always a celebrated miracle on day one," she writes. "Is it any less a miracle after sixty-three years?"

I walk a fine line, as a nurse, between saving lives and pissing people off. Jim's face is brick red. His neck veins bulge as thick as rat tails when he coughs. I'm elbow deep in frothy mucus, suctioning his tracheal stoma, the permanent breathing hole in his neck. The suction tube slurps the remaining juice with a satisfying *sloosh*. His coughing slows, and he blinks tears from his eyes. If his voice box hadn't been surgically removed, yesterday, a slew of profanities would escape him. Instead, he looks at me with eyes that teeter between *I hate you* and *Thank you*.

"How long have you been a nurse?" Jim's wife, Debby, asks from the other side of the hospital bed.

I'm tempted to answer, "First day on the job!" Her face is soft and flushed from her fear of having to learn to suction her husband's airway. She's up next. She buries her hands in the pockets of her cardigan as if she could make them disappear. I'll save that joke for another day.

I tell the truth. "Just over a year."

When I was fresh out of nursing school, a year ago, I would have hugged her. Part of me would like to, even now, but I know better. In school, nurses are taught to be gentle but professional. A nurse is to be poised, polite, and unbiased. A nurse is to love no patient but care for them all. Words like *empathetic* and *sympathetic* are discussed and debated so frequently that their meanings are tangled in my mind. No professor teaches ruthlessness to nursing students, yet after thirteen months on this unit, it's become second nature. It's not in the glossary of any guide to nursing interventions, but it's as important as any other skill. A good nurse must know how to attack.

I take a breath and brace myself. It's time to pick my first fight with Debby and Jim. "You're going to suction Jim's airway," I tell Debby, with no inflection of a question in my voice.

"Have you always wanted to work with head and neck cancer patients?" Debby asks. She shields herself from the strike with distraction.

Yes, while other little girls were dreaming of becoming movie stars, I was dreaming of dodging mucus bullets in a hospital room. Of course I didn't always want to do this! More than that, I never wanted to do it. I opt for selective honesty: "While in nursing school, I wanted to work in labor and delivery."

As a student, I dreamed of coaching soon-to-be moms as they brought their gooey, screaming babies into the world. I would hold the mom's hand, help her through labor, witness the miracle of life, clean that little miracle, and hand over the baby to the parents. Babies—pink and soft and new. I couldn't help but to love them. There was only one flaw in the plan: no job availability. So here I am on this postoperative unit, working with cancer patients who have had disfiguring and life-altering surgeries. My patients have had their eyes, tongues, ears, and noses surgically removed. They're real-life Mr. Potato Heads, a piece always missing. It's not the cozy blue-and-pink world of nursing in which I had envisioned myself. Instead of holding hands and instructing my patients to push, I'm pushing them to be independent, to let go of my hand.

"Labor and delivery?" Debby questions. "That's a whole different world!" I nod and hand her a 22-centimeter suction tube. I know her type. She'll talk for minutes, stalling, if I allow her. She pinches the tube between a finger and thumb, dangling it away from her body as if it's a slimy worm.

"Use both hands, like I showed you. Remember, you can't harm him." Jim's eyes spring wide with alarm, and I direct my comments to him. "Harming and hurting are different. She won't hurt you any more than I do."

"You get paid to hurt me!" Jim mouths. I laugh, unsure if he's joking. "I get paid to keep your airway from clogging up with mucus so you don't suffocate. You can't take me home with you next week, so you both must learn to do this."

"I really wish we could take you home!" Debby's voice bursts with longing. I stifle a laugh. She's not the first to request my services as a medical butler. Her shiny eyes focus on the quarter-size hole in his neck. It's the price he paid for the removal of his cancerous vocal cords. Also, for the reward of continued life. With the flashlight, we can see three inches down into the tunnel before the trachea curves. The surrounding skin is raw, swollen with sutures, and crusted with snot. "I can't do it." Her face scrunches up, on the brink of tears. She's never felt so vulnerable. She's never felt so helpless. I attack.

I force her hands into position on the catheter and shove them toward the hole. "I'm going to help you this first time," I say. That's what they want to hear, that you're the one in control. The part I leave out is that I'm going to let go, like a first ride without training wheels. Tough love. It's the only way.

We're nine centimeters into the trachea when I instruct Debby to press the suction gauge and begin swirling the tube around. Jim coughs from the agitation, and yellow froth spits out onto his chest hairs. Debby looks directly at Jim's face, thereby committing the cardinal sin of learning to suction your loved one. His features are contorted in pain, like a cartoon character being strangled. Her focus drops like a bowling ball. Her eyes mirror his panic, and she freezes, a deer in headlights.

"Don't stop! Swirl!" I demand.

"I'm stealing his oxygen!" she squeals. No, she isn't. I have already promised her that this is impossible. But in this moment when I set her free, adrenaline and emotion ricochet off the walls in the hospital room. It's complete pandemonium. Anything is possible, in her mind. She could go too far and jab his lung, stop his breathing altogether, even suck out his soul with that damned suction tube.

"Swirl!" I order.

Her wrist jerks in a frenzied side-to-side motion. One thing is missing: the *sloosh* sound of the mucus being sucked up through the tube. She's completely let go of the suction gauge. She whips the catheter out with blood-red cheeks, wild eyes, and a hint of breathless triumph.

In nursing school, I was taught to reassess after an intervention. Was the goal met? Yes or no? Success or failure? Debby did not, in fact, suction the airway. She also did not faint. It was really the most I could hope for on the first time.

"Perfect!" I say. More selective honesty. I'm sure that *something* about her effort was, indeed, perfect. I can't take the time to figure out exactly what. I'm a nurse, for God's sake; I have charting to do.

Jim gives a last hacking cough. A mustard-yellow snot rocket cannonballs out of his neck and splatters onto his white linen sheet. Debby looks to me for a reaction.

I smile encouragingly. "That's nothing. I've seen those suckers hit the wall. That's why we always stand to his side while we suction." She takes one look at the distance between her husband's neck and the wall, about ten feet, and turns too pale for my comfort. I pull up a chair. "Sit down. You've earned it." I know when to pull back. I'm an occasionally ruthless nurse, not a drill sergeant.

Jim glares at his wife with more of the *I hate you* and less of the *Thank you* in his eyes.

"You're doing great, Jim." I place my gloved hand on his shoulder. "Each day will get better. I promise." He nods his head and closes his eyes.

I turn my attention to Debby. "Really awesome job! I knew you could do it!" I cheerlead. "The more you suction him, the easier it will be. You'll be a pro in no time." If she doesn't become a pro, she will at least learn to suction during the suctioning process, but that's my secret to keep. For now she needs to soak in the victory of success to build her confidence. She deserves it.

My pager vibrates inside my scrub pocket, and I walk next door where a green call light is blinking over the doorframe. Roger raises his creaky body from the stiff visitor's chair. "Can I trouble you for some juice? I think my sugar is low." Roger is the husband of my patient, Rose. He's tall and thin with symmetrical features. I imagine he was attractive, years ago, before that demon leech named Old Age latched onto him and began to slowly drain his life.

"You're no trouble at all!" I wave a hand at him. "Sit down, and I'll be right back."

When I reenter with juice, Roger is hovering over Rose, suctioning out her tracheal airway as I taught him three days ago. He's a fast learner and good with his hands, which I attribute to his lifetime spent as a farmer. I wish Rose would fare as well. She's been mostly lifeless since surgery. There was no indication of stroke. The doctors say she's just not fighting. Giving in. Playing possum, if you will.

Roger is at her side day and night. He is my true patient. Rose is a body in a bed, and for her I am the robot nurse I was taught to be. Assessing, tasking, gentle, but not overly compassionate. Roger, however, has worn a soft spot in my heart. For him, I am human. He wets gauze with saline and begins to wipe Rose's neck where her incision seeps pink drainage. If this were Debby performing Jim's incision care, I would leave the room to chart.

"Let me get that for you," I say. "You sit down and drink up."

In our exchange, the straw is dropped and rolls under the bed. Roger bends to retrieve it. I can almost hear his spine and knees scream in protest. "No! I've got it!" I drop to my knees, but he stays right beside me.

"It was my own fault. I'll get it." His voice is gruff and determined. I am horrified as he sinks, lower, onto all fours to retrieve the straw. It's within my grasp, but I can see he needs this moment. I allow him to have control of this one small thing. Having solved that problem, he pulls himself up and takes a seat next to his wife, whom he cannot fix.

I do not promise Roger that every day will get better.

I ask him about his farm, his grandchildren, and the tattoo on his forearm. I won't remember his answers, but this room needs to be brightened with sounds of life, if only for a few minutes. I bathe Rose and change her Depends despite Roger's protests that he can take care of it. The room falls quiet while I work through my tasks. Roger has fallen asleep in the chair. It's a sad quiet, but a peaceful one. As I crush medication to put in Rose's feeding tube, Roger's voice breaks the nothingness in my head.

"Are you doing anything fun after work tonight?"

I laugh, caught off guard by his question. "After a twelve-hour shift, sitting on my couch with a novel is all the fun I can handle."

"Ah, youth is wasted on the young, they say." He rubs his hands over his bony knees. Our eyes connect. His are foggy blue over brown, a result of his cataracts, and glossy with fatigue. They open wider for a moment, clear and yielding truth. "Getting old sucks." The three words fly across the room and pierce my heart. They travel from right atrium to ventricle to lungs, and I can't breathe. Left atrium to ventricle to limbs, and I feel weak. I'm acutely aware of every miserable thing in this hospital room: the lifeless body, slack and pale; the ripe odor of fungal infection under layers of baby powder; the clicking machines feeding fluid into her nose and veins. All the things to which I'm conditioned to be numb jump out at me. My neck flashes with heat. For three fleeting heartbeats of a moment, I think I might cry. I pity Roger, yes, but equal to that—or perhaps more so—I fear becoming him.

"I think I'll stretch my legs," he announces as he always does before taking a lap around the unit.

Feeling disturbed, I shut the door and approach Rose; I lean in close. "Rose!" I hiss in a whisper. "Listen to me. Are you faking it? Rose! You need to open your eyes and get out of bed soon, or you'll grow too weak. If you're going to choose life, you need to hurry up and do it, already. Or else."

Or else death. As usual, Rose is unresponsive. No surprise there, but maybe she heard me. Advocating for patients and threatening them with the truth can be one and the same. Of course, I never read this in Bedside Manner 101, but maybe I'll write out my own rules of nursing, one day.

A few hours later, I'm changing out the linen basket in Jim's room when his very pregnant daughter waddles in. Helium balloons float from one hand. "Happy number sixty-three, one day early, Daddy!" She kisses him on the forehead. "How's it going today, Mom?"

"I suctioned Dad!" Debby blurts, rising to her feet. "Three times so far today!"

The daughter looks to me with disbelief, and I nod my head in affirmation. "*My* mother, who didn't like to clean the blood from our scraped knees? That's a miracle!"

"Why don't you explain the process to your daughter? See if you remember the steps," I suggest.

Ms. Timid transitions into Ms. Take Charge. "OK. Well, you always stand to the side of him so he doesn't cough up that gunk on you." She says it like she's said it a hundred times. The daughter crinkles her nose. "It's impossible to steal his oxygen, even though his face will turn red." Of course she remembers this time around. I listen to her full explanation before adding my two cents.

"His nurse wants to work in labor and delivery one day," Debby tells her daughter, nodding at her protruding belly.

"Babies versus Dad. I can't imagine you plan to stay on this unit for long. I mean, there's no common thread." The daughter is blunt. I feel a small ache at the thought of little newborns with their wrinkly feet.

I remember the first birth I witnessed as a student. The mother's fear. Her clenched teeth. The screaming. The father's bewilderment. His hands, which couldn't stay still. The dancing green line on the monitor that measured contractions. My counting out loud as I coached the mother to push. The doctor pulling the baby out and holding the little girl in the air like she was a trophy. The splash of surprise on the mother's face, as if she didn't truly believe there was a tiny person inside of her until it appeared. My cheeks were wet with tears, and I was embarrassed for crying. When the doctor looked at me, he gave me a knowing smile and said, "Amazing, right?" As I left the hospital that day, I walked through the parking lot with my heart full and pounding. The summer sky was blue and heaven twinkled above me, unseen. One day, I would get paid to do that. Deliver babies. Witness brand-new life, straight from God. I laughed out loud to myself. How lucky was I?

Obviously, that hasn't happened yet. Maybe it never will. Maybe that's OK with me. I'm still figuring it out.

"Your dad is kind of a big baby, so it's not entirely different," I tease. The mother and daughter hoot. Even Jim cracks a smile. "I need to get back to the nurses' station for shift change."

Nursing isn't what I pictured as a student. Caring isn't always about holding someone's hand. At the end of the day, I know I've done my job when my patient wants to let go of me. The harder I fight for Jim and Debby to be independent now, the better off they'll be in the end. Nursing surgical cancer patients isn't so different from nursing a newborn. Life is always a celebrated miracle on day one; is it any less a miracle after sixty-three years? And when a scary and disfiguring surgery buys new life, is that day any less special? More special? It's different. Miracles aren't always awe inspiring. They aren't always beautiful and obvious. Sometimes they're sticky and gross. Sometimes they're painful and full of loss. Sometimes you'll miss them if you blink. My eyes are wide open today.

"Wait," the daughter calls out. I turn at the door. "Dad's asking if you'll be his nurse again tomorrow." Jim looks at me with bushy eyebrows raised.

"You're stuck with me for a little while yet," I answer.

He winks and nods his approval.

"Don't think I'm taking it easy on you tomorrow because it's your birthday. You're going to learn to suction your airway." *Because you're lucky*, I think to myself. *Because you're able. Because you beat cancer. Because you were granted a new life, and you're going to take better care of your body the second time around, if I have anything to do with it.*

His wife smirks. "If I did it, you can do it."

He pouts his lower lip.

With my jacket on and keys in hand, I pass Rose's room. Roger sits with his chin resting on his chest. I knock lightly on the open door, and his gray face rises to mine.

"You headed out for the night?" he asks.

"Yeah. I was thinking you ought to do the same. Go home tonight and get a good night's rest. The pull-out beds are lousy."

He sighs. "Nah, I'm good here with Rose." I give him a tight-lipped smile. No use in arguing.

"I wish you'd take care of yourself like you take care of her," I say. "I worry about you."

"You're a good girl," he tells me. "You're a good nurse."

• • •

Am I? Maybe Roger is right to say so, but he told me I was a good person, first, and for me this is a valuable distinction. I have a lifetime of learning ahead of me. I apply many of the things I learned in school, but I've forgotten most. Random snippets of the rules come back to me, at times, but my mind will eventually eradicate them all, relearn them, and reinvent them. I remember two rules that always seemed tricky. First, a good nurse is unbiased. Yet, there's a universal rule that you don't choose who you love. Even strangers in a hospital room can steal your heart as quickly and easily as dropping a straw. Second, there's a difference between empathy and sympathy, and a good nurse solely empathizes. I haven't figured out how to be that sort of nurse, yet; honestly, I'm not interested in learning.

LAURA DEVANEY *has been an RN for four years and works on a radical head and neck unit in Indianapolis. She secretly favors patients who are old men because they always make her laugh. When she's not in scrubs, she writes young adult fiction.*

NEXT OF KIN

Josephine Ensign

Working at a clinic for the homeless in Richmond, Virginia, a nurse practitioner wonders whether she has become too friendly with a charismatic patient dying of AIDS. She asks, how close is too close?

On a cold April day in Richmond, Virginia, three years into my nursing career, I was attending a funeral for a patient. It was my first funeral of any sort. Standing at the graveside, I wondered why I had never been to one before. I was about to turn twenty-nine years old, and most people my age had surely been to a funeral. I wondered whether I should even be there—whether I had crossed so many professional lines that it was impossible to turn back.

The rain beat down hard and fast around me, sending its echoes under the canvas tarp and across the fields of tombstones. The words of the black Baptist preacher faltered, out of sync with the rhythm of the rain. He sucked in a lungful of biting air and led us in the Lord's Prayer. When he got to "and forgive us our debts," he straightened his spine and arched his neck backward, his eyes tightly closed and hands uplifted. A gray casket lay on a low table at his feet. Several flowered wreaths were strewn across its top, while some stood in front on spindly wire legs. A thin black woman sat in a metal folding chair near the casket. She wore a broad-brimmed black hat. A row of large black women stood behind her, the women like sentinels.

Approximately fifteen people huddled in clusters beneath the tarp—mostly women, a few uncomfortable-looking men, and one small boy in a fedora and an oversize raincoat, the sleeves hanging limply to his knees. He was fidgeting, pushing the hat back from his face, and twisting around to stare at me. I stood under the outer edge of the canvas tarp, one of the two white faces in the crowd and the only person not wearing black. I hadn't realized that people still wore black to funerals, and I felt embarrassed and worried that I was offending the family. The other white face belonged to an older social worker who was standing beside me; she had arranged the funeral.

I half-listened to the preacher as I tried to figure out the identity of the seated woman. Besides Lee, closed inside the casket, she was the center of this gathering; the preacher was more of a prop, like the flower wreaths. The social worker saw me gazing at the seated woman, leaned toward me, and whispered, "That's Lee's mother. He hadn't seen her in fifteen years. She got here too late."

I nodded and hugged my arms tighter, closing my coat. The wind had picked up and was blowing cold rain under the tarp. A gust toppled a flowered wreath. No one picked it up.

Lee was—or rather, he had been—thirty-eight years old, homeless, and a patient of mine for the past three years. I was repeatedly reminding myself that Lee was past tense. He had died of AIDS in the hospital the previous week, and now he, or at least his body, was in the casket and ready to be buried.

No, I shouldn't be here, I thought as I scanned the soft contours of the gray, wet graveyard. I felt my presence as an intrusion into this family's private and complicated grief for a side of this man that I hadn't witnessed.

There were ten or so parked cars lined up on the nearby road, and a large orange tractor revved its engine a few yards away to our left. It dangled a concrete casket encasement from its front, impatient to finish its business of burying Lee. I wondered if they were more respectful at private cemeteries. Lee was being buried in the potter's field section of the city-run Oakwood Cemetery; nearby was the all-black Evergreen Cemetery, its grounds overgrown with ivy, where human bones fell out of disintegrating mausoleums. At least this cemetery was well maintained, probably because of the roughly seventeen thousand Confederate soldiers buried here. Their graves were located near the entrance of the cemetery and were marked by short, white, and uniform gravestones, some adorned with small Confederate flags, that appeared to march over the hill. It struck me, for the first time, as more than an abstract idea that even in death are people divided.

As a nurse, I had seen death many times, had washed the newly dead at the hospital, done the paperwork, and zipped them into body bags. This was different. I was seeing where the body went after it left the body bag, the morgue, the funeral home. And I was seeing Lee's family for the first time. He had never mentioned them and did not ask for them in his final days. They were black, I was white, and we were in Richmond, capital of the Confederacy, where it's not easy to be colorblind. There were palpable barriers at the funeral: white and black; mother and son; healthcare provider and patient.

It was the spring of 1989, and I worked at a clinic in the Richmond Street Center—a multiservice, multiagency center for the homeless located in an old brick building on the edge of downtown and built on land that had at one time been the city dump. As a newly graduated nurse practitioner, I had been hired as the sole healthcare provider for the Street Center clinic, which was run by CrossOver Ministry, an evangelical Christian organization. A grant from The Sisters of Bon Secours paid my salary. I was neither Catholic nor evangelical, but I was married to a minister and called myself Christian. I held walk-in clinics twice daily during the week at the Street Center and performed outreach to patients residing in emergency shelters, under bridges, and by the river. On Saturday mornings, volunteer physicians came to the clinic to see the most medically complex patients. Patients like Lee.

As the preacher wrapped up Lee's graveside service with a final "Amen!" I thought over Lee's last year of life. He'd been diagnosed with advanced AIDS and disseminated tuberculosis—tuberculosis that was not only in his lungs but also in his spinal cord and bone marrow. I had helped to hold him still when the doctors had drilled a large needle into his hipbone for the marrow sample that would confirm the diagnosis. It was the only time I ever saw Lee cry.

He lived downstairs in the Street Center shelter for several months, spending his days with me in the clinic upstairs, where we had several exam rooms, a small waiting area, and a dental clinic used only on Saturdays. I gave him his daily medication injection and struggled to find enough remaining thigh muscle to accommodate the plunge of the two-inch needle. The medication was bright white and thick, the consistency of wet concrete. I dreaded giving him the shots, which seemed like acts of torture as I slowly squeezed the medication into his flesh. He never complained. After the shot, he'd swallow his other medications, curl up in the empty orange plastic dental chair, turn on the overhead exam lamp, and do crossword puzzles between naps. I'd throw an old army blanket over his shriveled form. Near the end of the clinic day, he'd emerge from the dental room, roll himself around the waiting room on an exam stool, laugh, and greet people in his affable, goofy way. Lee knew how to make me laugh. He appointed himself the clinic jester; he told me not to take things so seriously.

I *was* taking things seriously. I had an infant son and my marriage was ending. I was trying to extricate myself from a cliché affair with a married doctor whom I had met while taking care of Lee. I had lost my faith and was involved in a standoff with my boss, a conservative Christian minister who wanted me to return to my marriage and my church. He insisted I push patients like Lee to confess how they had gotten AIDS, push them to come back to Jesus before they died. I refused all these things. Within six months, I had lost my job, lost my home.

I was terrified that Lee's daily injections would lead to my becoming infected with HIV from a contaminated needle. I knew he already felt like an outcast, a leper, an Untouchable, so I usually tried not to wear gloves while I worked with him; but I wore two pairs when I gave him shots. By then, we mostly knew how the HIV virus was spread, but we had no medicine to prevent its transmission in the event of an accidental needle stick. After I'd been stuck by a needle the year before, I stopped nursing my infant son until I had confirmed that the patient was HIV negative. I still wasn't sure how far I'd go, how much I'd risk in the name of compassion or healthcare duty.

Soon after Lee had finished the month-long series of injections and was able to take medications on his own, I got a phone call.

"Nurse Jo, you got to come get me out of this place—talk to them and tell them I'm not crazy!"

The police had picked him up in nearby Monroe Park because he was talking loudly to himself and dancing around barefoot on frozen grass in November.

"Where are you—have you been taking your pills?" I grabbed some scrap paper and dug for his medical chart in a file cabinet; I quickly scanned his medication list, which had grown to several pages.

He hadn't been taking the medication that prevented the swelling around his brain from causing hallucinations. The police had escorted him to a small, private hospital up the street from the Street Center, and Lee was calling from the locked psychiatric ward where he was being held for observation. The doctors had committed him, against his will, to an inpatient psychiatric unit because they considered him a threat to himself or others—I wasn't sure which, since he'd been in a park acting crazy and probably scaring people. Legally they could hold him for observation for forty-eight hours, but on the second day, he was entitled to a hearing with a court magistrate who would decide whether or not to release him.

I arrived at the hospital to testify at his hearing the following morning. From the lobby, I had to take a special elevator, like the ones that grant access to the penthouse floor in an upscale hotel, which stopped only on the seventh-floor psychiatric unit. A secret code made it work. It seems like people look at you funny when you ask to take the psychiatric floor elevator; even being around crazy people is stigmatizing. Once on the floor, I had to show my ID, sign in, and be escorted into the unit by a burly male nurse. Entry was through a heavy metal door. As it closed with a thud behind me, I felt the air sucked from the hallway I had stepped into. I swallowed my panic.

We walked down an empty corridor painted in that peculiarly putrid shade of hospital green and entered a sunny, overly warm conference room. Sitting around the rectangular table were four white, middle-aged men: two in dark suits and ties, two in white coats. The white coats, of course, were Lee's doctors, and the others were the court magistrate and his assistant. It was a corner room with ceiling-to-floor windows on two sides, the sun streaming in on the men clustered at that end. As I stood, trying to decide where to sit, I had to squint against the sun to look at them. The intense light made me feel as if I were being interrogated by the police. Guilty by association—guilty of being crazy and disturbing the peace.

"Nurse Jo, thanks for coming!" Lee was huddled in a chair close to the door.

"Of course I would come." I brushed his shoulder with my hand as I sat down beside him.

Lee was dressed in several layers of blue hospital gowns, surrounded by the vulnerable air that clings to them. When the magistrate began his questioning, Lee kept his head down, answering *yes* or *no* in a barely audible whisper. The hearing went quickly. The magistrate decided to release Lee with the provision that he continue his medications under my supervision. I had to sign a form to acknowledge my responsibility for Lee's care. Otherwise, the magistrate said, Lee was a public health threat. Lee returned to the Street Center that afternoon, carrying a white plastic hospital bag filled with things like blue, stretchy hospital slippers, a toothbrush, and pages of typed discharge instructions.

Soon after his hospital stay, Lee grew more tired and wanted a place of his own—a room of his own. The Street Center social worker helped him to find a low-rent room in a house in a decaying section of Jackson Ward near the clinic, around the corner from a lifesize bronze Bojangles dancing on stairs. Every day, Lee came back to the Street Center in the outreach van for a hot meal and medications. The driver told me he had to throw pebbles at Lee's second-floor front window to let him know he'd arrived. There was no doorbell. The driver had never been inside the house, and neither had the social worker.

Lee hadn't answered the van driver's pebbles for three days in a row, and since his social worker was on vacation, I decided to check on him. It was a cold, bright day in mid-December. I pulled up in my car to the address given to me by the van driver. The sidewalk, street, and the block of row houses—most with boarded-up windows, several in black-charred ruins— were all deserted: no people, no stray dogs or cats, not even a squirrel. No signs of life. Yet the emptiness, the stark sunlight, and the shadows gave the scene a haunting and lonely beauty that was evocative of an Edward Hopper painting.

No one answered the door when I knocked, and I looked around for pebbles to throw at the window, trying to decide which size wouldn't break the glass. The small square patch of dirt at the base of the front steps was bare except for a pile of frozen dog excrement, so I walked to a potholed area of the street where I found some pieces of gravel. I speculated whether I could get arrested for vandalism and hoped the police wouldn't cruise by.

After I threw the gravel and got no response, I walked to the street corner where the landlord's office was located. I explained who I was and something about the situation to the plump, black woman behind a desk marked Property Manager.

"Oh, that Lee! He's probably just coming down off a drunk." She sighed heavily while pushing herself from the chair, then cuffed a large metal ring of keys hanging on the wall.

"Come on, let's go see."

I followed her down the street. She walked fast, swaying side to side and breathing heavily.

She opened the front door of Lee's building to reveal a dark hallway, but she didn't try to turn on the lights. The building had no electricity. There was enough sunlight from the curtainless windows to faintly illuminate the living room, which was empty except for the fast-food paper bags, empty beer cans, and liquor bottles strewn across the floor. There seemed to be no people in the house. As I followed the woman upstairs, a piece of wooden railing fell off under my hand and clattered to the floor below, raising a puff of dust. I worried that I'd damaged her property, but she didn't seem to notice. I continued to climb the stairs, now concerned that I might fall through myself. A smell that I struggled at first to identify reached me: the sweet-sick smell of human decay, of putrid flesh.

We turned left at the top of the stairs and passed an overflowing toilet that reeked of human excrement—there was no running water in the place, either, I noted—and a room whose only occupant was a half-burned mattress on the floor. Still no people. The property manager was breezy, business-like; she did not seem to see, smell, or be concerned about anything in the house. I'd been under bridges and in homeless encampments in the mudflats by the river that were more fit for human habitation. How can someone live here, I wondered, and how does someone charge another person money for a place like this? Weren't there laws against this kind of thing?

She rattled the key ring at a closed door near the front of the house. "Lee, you in there?" She didn't knock but moved to fling the door open.

"Yeah. I'm here," we heard faintly from inside.

"OK. The nurse is here to see you." Then, turning to me, "I gotta get back to the office." As she disappeared down the stairs, she bellowed over her shoulder, "Now behave yourself, Lee! You hear me?" She didn't wait for his answer.

Lee was hunched over on a folding cot inside the door. The room was not a room but rather a walk-in closet with a small window. The cot, a paper bag, and a small kerosene heater were all that fit in the space. Lee looked up at me with his dark eyes. His face was ashen. On the floor between his feet was a yellow hospital basin, half-filled with frothy pale-pink spit. Lee's breathing was so fast and shallow that he could barely speak.

"I wondered—when—you'd get here," he panted, grinning up at me.

"Lee, you look like hell. When did it get this bad?" I stalled for time, thinking that I'd have to call an ambulance, which meant that I needed to go back to the office of the property manager, whom I didn't want to see again, to borrow her phone. I wondered how black people could prey upon other black people, a thought followed by my awkward realization that this was a naïve and racist assumption. Still, I didn't want to see her again, and I felt indignant that she was part of a system that allowed people to live like this.

Lee refused an ambulance, complaining of the mounting medical bills he couldn't pay. I didn't point out that he wouldn't live long enough for the bills to matter; that seemed cruel. Instead, he let me take him to the medical college hospital in my car. I whisked his wheelchair into the emergency department and insisted he be seen right away, saying he was in respiratory distress—I used medical code words and knew I was being labeled as a troublemaker by the jaded staff. I was wearing jeans, a sweater, and a coat, but no lab coat or nametag that identified me as a healthcare professional. I knew how hospitals worked, this one especially since it was where I had gone to nursing school. I had done my share of labeling patients and their families. But they let us bypass the waiting room, and Lee was admitted to a medical unit for oxygen supplementation and a medical workup to see what was causing his respiratory distress.

Getting too close to my patients was something I had been taught to avoid. Healthcare providers are supposed to maintain a healthy emotional distance: a distance that prevents us from becoming so overwhelmed by our emotions that our provision of proper healthcare is crippled; a distance that prevents the professional burnout to which nurses are prone. It sounds good in theory, but there's no way to teach the location of that boundary to someone else, or to know where it is for yourself. There's no Berlin Wall or Rubicon River to clearly mark the divide. The business of nursing brings us into the messy swampland of human suffering, illness, and death. It is impossible to erect walls or channel rivers within a swamp. *Healthy emotional distance*—what does that mean in such terrain?

When I visited Lee the following day, the nurses asked me to help him fill out the consent forms that specified which procedures he wanted when he could no longer breathe on his own: did he want only comfort measures, or did he want to be put on a breathing machine? They handed me the forms and left us alone. By then, Lee knew he probably wasn't getting out of the hospital. He told me he was tired of being ill, so he signed the Do Not Resuscitate form. I wasn't sure if I had been neutral enough when I had explained it to him. I didn't want him to suffer. I knew there were worse things than death. After he signed the forms, he told me he wanted a chocolate milkshake from his favorite fast-food place. He smiled through his oxygen mask. I first had to finish some work at the clinic, and by the time I returned with the milkshake, Lee was in the intensive care unit and hooked up to a mechanical ventilator. The nurses told me that Lee's breathing had worsened to the point where he couldn't talk, and when asked whether he had changed his mind about the consent forms, he nodded yes. I was dubious, but I hadn't been there. Nor did I know how it felt to slowly suffocate. It crossed my mind that this was a teaching hospital, and perhaps the doctors wanted to prolong Lee's life— teaching fodder for young physicians. I pushed these thoughts away.

Lee went quickly into a coma, his temperature spiking close to 110°F, higher than I'd known was possible. They placed Lee's bloated but emaciated body on a blue ice pad atop an air mattress, whose noisy sucking mingled with the softer sighs of his ventilator.

He lingered in that state for days, then for over a week. His medical team finally called for an ethics committee meeting to decide whether he should be disconnected from the machines that kept him alive, lingering neither here nor there. They asked me to be at the meeting. I found myself in another hospital conference room with his doctors and the hospital chaplain. The Street Center social worker had been trying to find Lee's family members ever since he was first hospitalized, but none had been located. I sat at one end of the conference table. Lee's senior doctor was droning on, reciting dry medical facts about Lee's case in a precise, organized manner, looking up from his notes to the ceiling and back down again, as if lost in a soliloquy.

They discussed Lee's case for a half hour, at the end of which his medical team voted to stop the machines the next day. I was relieved they didn't ask me to vote, but they did ask me what I thought he would want. I told them he was tired of being ill, and if he couldn't get better, he wanted to die.

After the meeting, I went back to Lee's bed behind the white curtain that separated him from other critically ill patients. He was alone in his curtained space. I touched his burning hand and said a silent good-bye.

I stood at the end of his bed, contemplating what else to do, wondering what was proper in a situation like this. Do you just say good-bye and leave, or do you say something profound and make solemn promises like "Lee, I will make sure no one ever dies like this again"? Wasn't that a bit grand and narcissistic? But that's what I said.

Not wanting to leave too hastily, I glanced around the room. His aluminum-clad medical chart hung from a rack at the end of his bed. Curious what the hospital knew about Lee that I didn't, I grabbed the chart and quickly scanned it from the back forwards: results of numerous blood tests, recordings of Lee's vital signs, and pages of nurses' notes with entries such as "patient resting comfortably" written in flowery cursive. On a typed intake form, the first page of the chart, I noticed my name beside the category Next of Kin. My first reaction was shock that the hospital staff had made such a mistake: how could a Nordic-looking white girl like me be this black man's next of kin? I closed the chart and hung it back in its rack before the nurses could come in and scold me. But I now knew I'd gotten too close to this patient of mine. Lee and I were bound by something like blood.

I've been a nurse for almost thirty years. I didn't burn out. I crossed professional lines early in my career, and they got me here—to the sublime swampland of living.

I visited Lee again in early October 2011, at the cemetery where he'd been buried over two decades earlier. It was a bright fall afternoon, warm and windless, and I needed help to find him. A woman in the cemetery office pulled the crumbling leather-bound ledgers from a large fireproof safe and looked up the location of his unmarked grave; it was in a section now called Social Services.

"He's in the old section. I'll have to get someone to take you back there or you'll never find it," she said, smiling at me through layers of fake-gold jewelry.

The gravedigger was a graying black man, taciturn. He looked quizzically at me when I told him I was looking for my friend. In my Dodge Avenger rental with New Jersey license plates, I followed the gravedigger's battered truck, the bed of which was filled with red clay and shovels. We crossed a ravine, a stream, a marsh. He led me to a wide, flat field without headstones and paced a few steps from a metal grave marker he found covered by grass.

"Here he is. This here's his head."

"How can you tell?"

"They're buried every five feet, heads away from the road. And they sink in. See, like here," he said, pointing to a large depression. "I have to keep fillin' 'em up with dirt. It's clay here, mostly—not good for burying."

I thanked him and said I wanted to stay and talk with my friend. He nodded and drove away. I was alone. No one was walking or driving in the back section of the cemetery.

Lee's grave was covered with freshly mown weeds—dandelions and crabgrass. Gazing across the expanse of unmarked graves, listening to the sound of crickets, I did not feel like I was in a field of despair. As I walked across the grass, I almost fell into a dark, two-foot-wide hole at one of the graves. I laughed, wondering how I would explain an injury from such an accident. There was a stone bench to one side of the field, near the road. Dated 1990, it was inscribed: To our homeless sisters and brothers. Be at peace. I recognized the names of other patients of mine on a few of the scattered flat grave markers. I realized that Lee was surrounded by his friends, his drinking buddies, his homeless family. He was at home. I didn't try to talk to him or make promises this time, but I left some wild asters on his grave.

JOSEPHINE ENSIGN *teaches health policy at the University of Washington in Seattle. Her literary nonfiction essays have appeared in* The Sun, Oberlin Alumni Magazine, *and* Silk Road. *She is writing a book,* Catching Homelessness, *a narrative nonfiction account of her work as a nurse practitioner who provided healthcare to homeless people while navigating her own passage through homelessness. She writes a blog,* Medical Margins, *on health policy and nursing.*

HEALING WANG JIE'S BOTTOM

L. Darby-Zhao

Medical supplies are lacking where a nuse heeding a call to service works in rural China. One patient's survival may depend on resilience, a tight-knit family, and a salve made from white sugar and pear blossom honey.

The bedsore and I got to know one another in an oddly decorated bedroom on the outskirts of a disheveled Chinese village. It was a rocky relationship from the start. The thing about bedsores, as you might know, is that they often turn out to be much deeper than they first appear. This is a lovely quality to find in a man. In a bedsore, not so much.

I had to travel to reach the village. Plane, bus, taxi, train. I strung the machines together like big metal beads, groggily alighting from one and duly boarding the next. I used them in a descending order of technological complexity, first crossing oceans, then bisecting the sallow countryside of northern China. Decades of hard-won economic developments seemed to happen in reverse, like a propaganda film screened backward on the train car's grimy windows, as I headed south from the Beijing–Tianjin area. I bumped down Maslow's hierarchy and landed, briefly stunned, in the courtyard of a mud-and-brick home near the bottom. The final few meters to the house were covered by foot. Ah, feet.

I had completed my final exhausting twelve-hour shift on the pediatrics unit of a well-funded, well-stocked teaching hospital in the Washington, DC, metropolitan area several months earlier. Located in Fairfax County, Virginia, which consistently ranks as one of the richest counties in America, the hospital was extremely handsome in that well-groomed, suburban sort of way. It had the requisite cappuccino cart in each lobby and Starbucks on tap in the cafeteria, amenities of which I availed myself daily, yet hypocritically disdained.

My gravely ill, fully insured little patients; my talented, highly motivated nursing colleagues; the adorably disoriented interns; the round-the-clock pediatric residents; the conscientious attending physicians; the specialist consultants—over the course of a beeper-interrupted afternoon farewell party, they became characters from my past. They had been entwined with my everyday life; we even breathed the same contaminated air during the annual respiratory syncytial virus epidemic. One of the charge nurses mused that she hadn't realized how popular I was with the doctors until she asked them to sign my card; they all expressed genuine sadness at my departure. And why wouldn't they miss me? I was so eager to please and so very conscientious. I was a total suck-up. Unlike those staff nurses who craved more autonomy, who were frustrated by their positions in the chain of command, who aspired to be pediatric nurse practitioners or nurse anesthetists, I loved taking orders. I actually *enjoyed* taking, following, and (especially) signing off on physicians' orders. I probably had not quite thought this through when I heeded the call to service in rural China, where there were no orders to follow.

The bedroom ceiling was the only thing Wang Jie had seen for weeks. She lay supine, twenty-four hours a day, staring at it. I'm no Dr. Gregory House, but the cavernous bedsore that had developed on her sacrum, at the base of her spine, just might have been related to this situation. Her ceiling was hand-woven from an advertisement for local brand of laundry detergent, forming a surface like a picnic basket lid. It kept Wang Jie contained, her body slowly starting to spoil from one mushy spot. About ten copies of the same large poster had been cut into strips surely with iron scissors, standard issue in rural Chinese households and which have huge handles seemingly designed to fit the paws of a large panda. Each bit of the model's face, body, and clothing had been sliced to pieces. The pattern of the weave allowed no complete image to be seen at a glance, but if one studied the ceiling long enough, the scattered body parts could be mentally arranged back into wholeness. There was something addictive about it. Wang Jie, I assumed, had done this a thousand times over.

When I crossed the dusty courtyard to meet her for the first time, I found Wang Jie motionless except for the newly atrophied arm she lifted weakly in greeting. She was resigned and inert, her body pressed onto the *kang,* a sleeping platform made of heated brick, and held there by layers of musty, cotton-filled quilts. I understood later that she was very much an emotional and psychological shutin, as well, that her assessment of her circumstances was defined by her belief in *ming,* which cannot be adequately translated into English. My mother-in-law, who lost her adolescence, her education, and her aspirations to the chaos of the Cultural Revolution, says simply— though always with a sigh—that this was her ming. It is a belief in fate with a Chinese twist, and Wang Jie's ming held her in place as firmly as her thoracic-level spinal injury did.

This meeting among Wang Jie, her bedsore, and me, the naïve pediatric nurse, came about partly because of my tendency to make big decisions quickly, move forward ingenuously, and hope for everything to work out for the best. I had majored in English literature, trying out five different minors before settling on Biblical literature (with just enough time to complete the credits), then switched gears after graduation and got myself a nursing degree. I promptly landed a staff nurse position in pediatrics, finished up an internship at my church, and left for China three years later. Under the instruction of some brilliant teachers, Mandarin Chinese came to me quite easily, and I was soon declared linguistically competent for charity health work, as planned. They had all worked out so nicely, my choices.

For Wang Jie, in whose half-paralyzed body the decubitus ulcer grew, this meeting was about the conspicuous absence of choices. She had not chosen to live her entire life in Qing County, which, I can attest, having traveled the country widely, has one of the least appealing natural landscapes in China. The years I worked in Qing County were plagued by drought, and the one remaining river was so polluted with runoff from a nearby paper factory that the stinking water flowed dark purple, murky and opaque. One expected to see the kids who played in its waters dyed the hue of ripe little eggplants. In ancient times, Qing County was called Gan-ning. While *ning* implies tranquility, *gan* means dry, or hollow, and when we use it in common speech, it carries a connotation of helplessness, of one's efforts having all been in vain.

Neither had Wang Jie any choice in regard to her arranged marriage to Li Ge, her first cousin, which had shifted her identity from farmer's daughter to farmer's wife with one stamp of the official red *zhang*. She'd had no choice but to grow dates and apples, as opposed to some other crop, and no choice but to go to market to sell her husband's apples on that particular day. No choice about the old and unsteady three-wheeled farm truck she rumbled over the ramshackle bridge, its guardrails long gone, its crumbly cement surface uneven and waiting for just such a convergence of factors. With one unfortunate turn of the wheel, she tumbled ten meters down to the dry riverbed, where her vertebrae piled up like compartments in a commuter train crash.

Wang Jie had been discharged from—or rather, she just sort of left—the hospital closest to her village several weeks before I met her. Although some progress in rural health policy has been made over the past few years, at the time there was no medical insurance or government subsidy available to someone in her situation. To be admitted to the hospital, to be even physically allowed inside, the family of a patient who had been involved in a major accident like Wang Jie's had to first hand over a minimum of ¥3,000, two to three years' farming income, which was then equivalent to about $360. This amount was obviously burdensome, and this was only the beginning. Cash, and lots of it, had to be rounded up from relatives, fast. I helped with other cases over the years and was surprised every time by the sight of apparently destitute farmers who suddenly produced enormous wads of grubby bills, literally from under their mattresses, to cover the medical expenses of their siblings, parents, and the random relatives whom Westerners would consider distant kin but whom the Chinese consider close family connections. This is the system.

Wang Jie's doctors had inserted a urinary catheter and taken an image of her crumpled spine with their behemoth X-ray machine, which must have been forged in someone's backyard during the Great Leap Forward. Honest to God, I have no idea what they did for her after that. The extended family had lent them about ¥40,000. I never got a clear account from either Wang Jie or Li Ge (who was being treated for a shattered ankle) of the treatments that this sum, more than enough to plunge them into debt for the rest of their lives, paid for. I realized later that they probably didn't quite know either. What I do know is that none of it went to nursing care, since there are no nurses in the low-level rural medical centers. Instead the junior doctors begrudgingly assist the patient's family, which performs a portion of what we would consider nursing duties. The rest of the stuff in my bulky western protocol manuals was not even dreamed of. When Wang Jie left the hospital, she hadn't been moved from her supine position, been bathed, had a bowel and bladder program initiated, or received wound care. She had received no instruction but to avoid drafts, which is the first tenet of Chinese medical advice for every ailment. In her village of Lixingcun, as in all the villages, there were no visiting nurses, no physical or occupational therapists, and no doctors qualified to give follow-up care to a new paraplegic.

Thus, it was due to an utter lack of other options that I was called on to help. In China, former classmates are the number one source for professional contacts, the second is family, and the third is drunken banquets. A few years before Wang Jie would stay in the hospital, its director feted someone from my charity organization. Amid the smoke and general dissipation, the director obtained my supervisor's cell number; when he sought assistance for Wang Jie, he rang the number, and the call was forwarded to me. Although I was on the medical team, I was, in some ways, the least of the last resorts, a scraping from the bottom of the healthcare barrel in terms of both skill and cultural awareness. The language barrier (my celebrated Chinese crashed and burned in the sea of aural torment that was the Qing County dialect), my lack of adult rehab nursing experience, and the distance of the village from my home base in Tianjin—not to mention my slowness to develop a taste for whiskey-soaked red dates and hand-rolled cigarettes the size of dachshund puppies— were all formidable obstacles. For once in my life, I demurred. But Wang Jie was a patient in need of care, and when you're dealing with a reluctant—but ultimately compassionate and eager to please—nurse, that's your trump card.

So I found myself in Wang Jie's bedroom, poking a homemade paste of pear blossom honey and coarse white sugar deep into her labyrinthine pressure ulcer with—what else?—chopsticks. Her diminutive thirteen-year-old daughter, Xiao Hua, rolled her mother onto her right side while I crouched on the kang, David Werner's *Disabled Village Children* propped open beside me. This incredibly useful book not only explains the antibiotic and healing properties of honey and sugar for pressure sores (who knew!), but also teaches things like how to make a walker entirely out of wood (including the wheels!) and, my personal favorite, a baby rattle from a cow's horn. The book doesn't tell you how surprised you'll be when this stuff actually works.

I taught Xiao Hua how to debride the wound, rinse and replace the honey paste three times per day, and change her mother's position every two hours, always keeping the pressure completely off the wound. Wang Jie's obliterated tissue was thus coaxed back into existence, cell by beautiful cell. Wang Jie and I were amazed, not to mention totally impressed with ourselves. I felt as though we were creating it ex nihilo, her brand-new flesh. For Wang Jie, each reappearing bit of her body was another step toward her defiant victory over the abysmal long-term survival rate for paraplegics in the Hebei Province villages.

Those were the frustrating days of hopeless dial-up Internet in the Tianjin dorms, where I lived, and the death trap web cafés that made international news when they caught fire, their doors held shut with bicycle locks, while stuffed full with students. With no reliable Internet access, I had only my nursing textbooks, which I had lugged halfway around the world. On my days off, my curiosity compelled me to research the sort of nursing care I would have given to a well-off American bedsore. Apparently, I would have been culturing, measuring, and staging it, among other things, while wearing really cute scrubs. I realized that Wang Jie's wound, given her visible bone, had been a stage IV—the worst—when I had started treatment. While it was frustrating to know that proper nursing care would have prevented this dire situation from developing, or would have at least controlled it (even Christopher Reeve had bedsores), it was also satisfying to know that we were beginning to win this battle against such a formidable foe.

While we mounted our offense on and obsessed over the bedsore, I was also making sure to fixate on Wang Jie's other paralysis-related problems, which included the challenge of sitting her up for the first time. My sources scared me out of my wits with their dire warnings about extreme orthostatic hypotension and the related loss-of-consciousness-type catastrophes that can follow if the patient is positioned upright too quickly. I have never been good with unconscious patients since my main asset, a sparkling personality, goes somewhat underappreciated. So I put off the task of sitting her up because I was scared and no one was ordering me to do it. True to American nursing form, though, I eventually created a detailed plan for elevating Wang Jie's upper body, degree by degree, over the course of days. I may have even made a graph for the occasion. Wang Jie, however, made up her own mind, blew me off, and demanded to be sat up; with her family's assistance, the task was accomplished in one swift movement, causing *me* to almost pass out. She was perfectly fine.

The village received the wheelchair like King David received the Ark of the Covenant upon its return to Jerusalem. Perhaps there wasn't quite as much dancing or sacrificing of bulls, but surely there was the same perfect mixture of joy and awe in the air as we awkwardly unloaded the basic model wheelchair from the van. If I remember correctly, it was the only model available for purchase in Tianjin, a city twice the size of Chicago. We bought it with donations for about eighty bucks. By that time, I had organized Wang Jie's family into a multidisciplinary care team with Li Ge in charge of physical therapy. Under the tutelage of one of my physical therapist roommates, he took charge of teaching his wife kang-wheelchair transfers, as well as the more strenuous (due to the incline) wheelchair-kang transfers. Wang Jie's chair soon became the home's mobile command center.

Wei Hong, the sweet and perpetually embarrassed sixteen-year-old son, showed an aptitude for cooking and thus became his mother's nutritionist and dietician. Xiao Hua continued to grow in her roles as nursing assistant and de facto nurse. She had dropped out of school after the accident in order to care for her mother, a decision I tried to get her to reverse, to no effect. There are no alternative education options for kids who drop out of school in Qing County, and we all knew that once she started down that road, her chance for an education was over. But she was driven by loyalty, duty, and love; I, the foreign *ayi* with the irrelevant opinions, was no match. Xiao Hua, who I don't think managed to get even her middle school diploma, is made of tough stuff. I should have realized this when I taught her how to do her mother's urinary catheterization, which has caused many a nursing student to sweat and knock knees. Xiao Hua did it perfectly on the first try, without a flinch.

All of the healable parts of Wang Jie's body were slowly mending, she had wheels, and her family was becoming closer as its members cared for her and grew accustomed to their new circumstances. Wang Jie then decided it was time to deal with a couple other things that had been bugging her. First, she tackled and soundly defeated her illiteracy. Learning to read Chinese is a very laborious process, to say the least. There's no *Hooked on Phonics;* the thousands of *hanzi* characters must be memorized one by one. She wanted to be literate, she said, so she could write her name and her children's names and read the Bible. Qing County women have an OK literacy rate, for rural China, but Wang Jie had gone to school for only one year when she was six years old. The cause for her brief enrollment became clear when I met her highly unstable, hypochondriac mother. Li Ge made hanzi cards for her and glued them to the walls. She started with *wo* and *ni*—"me" and "you"—and didn't stop.

Then came the lawsuit. It's hard for me to imagine, after my time in Qing County, that lawyers actually exist there, and even more difficult to believe them capable of winning a case against the government. But they successfully sued the roads department of the local government for negligence and subsequently recovered the costs of Wang Jie's medical bills. It may have been unprecedented in Qing County. Wang Jie and Li Ge used the money to repay their relatives, which was actually a gift to their children; they stopped the cycle of debt that rolls down to the next generation when it is not repaid. Wei Hong and Xiao Hua were thus set free. Wei Hong is now a sous-chef at a big restaurant in the Tianjin suburbs. Xiao Hua is married and has given Wang Jie and Li Ge a fat little grandson.

Twelve years have passed since I boarded that plane and left my nursing job in America. I had loved pediatrics, had loved how peds nurses often took care of the parents, almost as much as the child, because a child's hospitalization is one of the most stressful events a family will ever encounter. I miss giving everything that I have—professionally, intellectually, emotionally, and physically—for twelve hours straight. I miss being so exhausted after a shift that I can't speak, can't even lift my arm to check the messages on my phone, can't do anything but sit in an old blue recliner, catatonic, watching reruns of *Law & Order*. I traded it all for a different type of nursing and a very different brand of exhaustion. My nursing exhaustion in China has been the consequence of never quite understanding everything that someone is saying; of always straining to catch the meaning within the meaning; of traveling hours back and forth on buses and trains that are standing room only, alternately freezing or sweltering; of not having the right supplies and not knowing how to say them, much less where to get them; not knowing if I am being helpful or being used.

I'm now back in touch with my old nursing colleagues. Or I've at least started to reconnect with them, when I can get around the Chinese government's Facebook restrictions. My friends have progressed and developed in their careers as nurses, real hands-on nurses, while my skills and interests have become broader, less clinical over the past few years. I can't remember the last time I listened to someone's lungs other than my daughter's. Do I regret it? There are pangs. When I've just spent hours writing project reports, which along with grant proposals are the foundation of all NGO drudgery, those pangs are sharp indeed. I would much rather be writing nursing notes, believe it or not. Then I'll get a call from Wang Jie. She is now the proud owner of Xiao Hua's old cell phone, and she uses it to periodically check in with me. She tells me about some hymns she's learned or how naughty her grandson is, and then reports, in much detail and in that Qing County dialect that is finally starting to grow on me, how she and Li Ge are keeping her bedsores well under control. In her eyes, I am still her nurse.

L. DARBY-ZHAO *has spent twelve years working on women's and children's health initiatives in China. She holds a master's degree in mother and child health from University College London.*

ZEITGEBER

Denise Elliott

For a night-shift nurse the pediatric intensive care unit (PICU) is a world often interrupted by life-threatening crises.

I.

It is only 7:00 p.m., but it is dark outside and snowing a bit. The roads were icy on my ride in. *Major trauma, impact with the side of the car seat.* I am not ready, nor do not I want to be. My mind goes to a dark place to hide while I carry on with a smile. How bad is it? *Who* is it? I pray it's no one I know. As in the child's game of telephone, information comes to night-shift nurses fourth, fifth, even sixth, hand; what we are told is rarely what arrives.

Flip on the lights in the empty room. Make a quick visual sweep of its contents, note the present equipment, as well as the absent things you'll need to bring in. Unlock the drawers of the medical supply cart and make sure the dividers in each drawer are properly stocked with gauze pads, various gauges of needles, diapers, alcohol wipes, and paper tape. Open the larger drawers and look for sterile saline, sterile water, tubing for oxygen.

Mentally check off things to consider: first, airway management. Remove and unwrap a package of oxygen tubing and attach the fluted end to the green, plastic oxygen port protruding from the wall. Open suction tubing and attach it to the red plastic port on the closed suction bucket that's connected to the suction outlet on the wall. Stack packages of intubation equipment, artificial airways, and emergency tracheotomy kits—tiny plastic tubes to be inserted into a patient's neck, allowing us to administer oxygen or institute artificial breathing with a resuscitation bag or ventilator. Check the resuscitation bag and place a new mask by its side.

Second, cardiac care. Bring over packages of new wire leads for monitoring the heart. Be sure to have leads of various sizes—infant, child, teen. Turn the monitor screen on and verify that it loads. Turn it off. Hang a paper sheet of check-off boxes in case there is a cardiac emergency. Hang an IV bag from which the nurses can draw fluids for medication administration. Hang an IV bag we can hook up to the patient. Bring the crash cart from down the hall and set it up outside the room.

Finally, the little things. Open the cupboards and verify that there is an adequate supply of sheets, towels, washcloths, and absorbent pads. Hang another checklist with little boxes to record admission details and any procedures that will be performed upon arrival. Look around the room again, satisfied that everything is in its place, that everything you will need is within arm's reach. Turn off the lights, take a deep breath, and wait.

The helicopter circles over the hospital, its blades chopping at the air and rattling the windows. It wakes the sleeping babies down the hall. Three cry out simultaneously, and nurses shuffle off to console them and shush them back to sleep. From the window of the empty room, I see the helicopter landing in the darkness, illuminating the giant red X painted on the roof. A medical team races toward it, heads bowed low, pushing an empty stretcher. The tiny bundle of patient is collected, strapped onto the stretcher, and followed into the building by the helicopter crew. Mouths are moving, but I cannot hear what they are saying. Fine snow coats the crew members hair and swirls around them like sparkling dust devils. I look around the room again, double-checking that every needed thing is here.

We are given phones when we come on the floor to work, and mine rings in my pocket; the trauma team assesses the patient's needs and updates us so the room can be prepared adequately. It will be a while before they arrive on the unit because they must first go through the pediatric emergency department for admission. I go to the storage room to get resuscitation equipment and a surgical tray for the line that will be inserted into an artery. Stock up on IV bags of normal saline—0.9 percent sodium chloride in sterile water, as close as you can come to the salinity of blood. Carry it all to the empty room.

The infant in room three is crying. I check her diaper and her leg, where her IV is inserted, ensure that all monitor leads are properly attached to her chest, and bundle her in a soft flannel receiving blanket. I still have time to hold and cuddle her before my trauma patient arrives. Her IV pump alarms. A quick look at the machine reveals that pressure is building up in the tubing. I gently adjust her tiny leg, where the IV runs beneath the blanket and into her vein. The line that monitors pressure on the pump recedes, its pressure reduced, and I place her sleepy body into the warm bassinette with the high-tech heater, positioning her on gel pads in order to prevent pressure sores. Now that she is quiet, I can check her vital signs with the tiny disposable blood pressure cuff. It hums and clicks, filling with a small amount of air. She straightens her leg against the intrusion and lets out a sharp cry of protest before settling again. The machine readjusts the pressure for an accurate reading. All is well and within normal limits. The resident pokes her head in the door to ask how she is. She walks over to the bassinette and takes one tiny hand in hers; the infant gives a reflexive squeeze. She listens to her chest, listens to my report, and makes her way to the next room.

There is a flurry of activity down the hall. I look at my watch; only fifteen minutes have passed. They made record time admitting this patient. The resident and four of the nurses on the unit join me. It will take that many, maybe more, to make the process go smoothly.

They are whispering that the child is already dead as they carry him, strapped to a blue trauma board, to the bed. They do not mean really dead—just brain dead. He was hypoxic, lacking adequate oxygen, for over an hour while receiving CPR en route. A tube is placed in his throat to aid his breathing, but it doesn't mean the oxygen will circulate well. Fluid has accumulated in the fibrous sac surrounding the heart, which won't stretch to accommodate the extra fluid. Unable to pump or move, the heart slows due to the pressure. It's like an overfilled water balloon about to burst. No blood circulates, no oxygen is carried to the body's tissues. An oscillatory ventilation machine is cycling at over one hundred breaths per minute, more than four times the normal respiratory rate for a healthy child of this size, and it's still not enough. The body has been cooled to prevent further damage from the lack of oxygen and shows a temperature of 29°C (84°F). The CT scan says it is too late. No one knows the child's name, and they refer to him as Trauma. Someone, somewhere knows his name, but it has been lost in the bustle.

Fluids are pushed directly into the bone of his leg through an intraosseous needle. A large-bore needle is inserted directly into the tibia, the long inner bone of the lower leg that starts at the knee and points toward the big toe.

The child arrived in blood-soaked sheets. I attach suction to a tube that extends through his nose and down his throat, and blood is sucked from his stomach. Blood pools in the catheter bag. Blood oozes out of every orifice. I move in a coordinated effort with the other four nurses, the resident, and the physician to provide medications and fluids, change tubing, insert IVs, manage the airway, and pump oxygen into the tiny lungs with an ambu-bag. We report any sounds we hear in the lungs. The respiratory therapist oversees the connection of a new ventilator and draws blood from an artery for an immediate evaluation of the body's systems. Oxygen-saturation levels, blood pressure, heart rate, and core body temperature are displayed, color-coded and flashing, on the monitors. A fifth nurse writes the numbers in the tiny boxes and calls them out if they change significantly in either direction; every injected, removed, or oozing drop of fluid is recorded. Whenever resuscitation medication is given, she writes it down, along with the immediate change (or lack thereof) in vital signs. Medical responses are regimented, recorded, systematic. A sixth nurse stands in the doorway, ready to run for supplies or equipment.

Masks and head coverings are handed out to prepare us for the insertion of an arterial line, a tube going directly into an artery that will more accurately monitor blood pressure. It will also allow us to remove blood for analysis, or to administer fluids and medications. It is a sterile surgical procedure; we do not want to contaminate the site with the germs we carry in our throats or hair, a strand of which could float down onto the sterile field. Blood work results are reported to the physician, who inserts the arterial line through the groin. He orders bicarbonate and more fluids to correct the acidic imbalance in the blood that has been created by ineffective breathing. Surgeons stand in the doorway, offering their expert opinions and reading X-rays that arrive on the room's portable computer.

The parents are held in the waiting area. They are anxious and unable to wait, and they wander down the hall to look in the window before a seventh nurse quickly ushers them back to the waiting area. The pediatrician whispers to no one in particular that the parents are not aware of the extent of the injuries. No one has told them yet.

A nurse from another unit arrives to care for patients on the floor while all the PICU nurses are busy with the trauma. After an hour of nonstop effort, the child has not been stabilized, and the physician states that there's little more we can do. The child's heart is still beating, but irregularly. The ventilator continues to force oxygen into the tiny lungs. His blood pressure swings wildly, and his core body temperature has been raised only by a degree or two, despite the electric warming blankets. A chaplain arrives. The pediatrician, surgeon, and chaplain take the parents into a quiet conference room to tell them the news.

Dad comes out of the conference room, tears flowing, his face red and contorted with grief. Mom comes out and cannot make it down the hall; she sits against the wall with her head between her knees, her body wracked by sobbing. The extended family starts to arrive, and Dad breaks down again. Mom is led to her child's room, unable to look up from the pile of tear-soaked tissues she holds tightly against her face. The family gathers around as the chaplain reads verses over the child.

Only another nurse and I are left in the room, weaving between family members and continually assessing the patient's status. Deliver fluids and medications. Do not make eye contact. Do not look at the child and compare the beautiful blond curls to those of your own child at home. Keep your head down and attend to the care routine. Fluff and straighten the sheets. Untangle tubing. Adjust the IV drip rate. You cannot leave the room because of the constant need for medications to be administered, fluids adjusted, the ventilator monitored, assessments made. Ignore your full bladder. Make notes in the boxes. The physician comes to the door and quietly informs us that the child's organs will be harvested at the request of the parents; like magic, the surgical team arrives to escort both patient and family to the operating room. With the physician and the surgical team, I step out to give the parents and family time alone.

Through the open door, we see the family collapse on the bed of the child, the mother trying to gather him in her arms; it's impossible because of the wires, the tubing, and the Bair Hugger machine's warm padding that has been expanded over his tiny body like giant bubble wrap. The chaplain is saying a prayer so loudly that the parents in other rooms close their doors and pull the curtains. They protect themselves and their children from the pain of the short-term guest. There is sobbing and wailing and family members leaning their heads against the cool walls, their tears flowing down the white paint and their hot cheeks, soaking their shirts and sweaters. The entire staff looks away.

After my trauma patient has been removed from the unit, room three wakes and cries. I gather her into my arms, careful of the tubing that extends from her body. I sit in the rocking chair by her bedside and feed her. She does not coo or open her eyes to look around, but I feel her warm body instantly relax the moment she's in my arms. She smells good, and I instinctively breathe her in. She finishes her bottle in a sleepy daze.

At 7:00 a.m., I give my report to the same nurse whom I relieved last night. Like every morning, I put on my coat and walk to my car. Brush the snow off the windshield, sit in the seat, put the key in the ignition, start it. Unlike every morning, my entire body shakes with grief. It is a full ten minutes before I gather myself for the drive home. Back up the car, drive out of the parking lot, and slowly make my way home on the icy, dark, and desolate roads.

II.

The cold night air has a particular smell. Deep and almost musty, it is tinged with the scent of the darkest dirt under the forest's frozen leaves. It carries the essences of frozen bark and the crispy, long-dead seed heads of black-eyed Susans picked over by birds and mice. The neighbor's wind-chimes *ting-ting-ting* as I sip hot coffee and listen to my breath, my thoughts. Sleep never comes at night anymore; the night shift claimed my circadian rhythm long ago. The house, claustrophobic in its nighttime hush, forces me outside to wait for the sunrise—the signal that it's time to sleep.

III.

The floor is sleepy, and a hush falls as the lights are lowered in the halls and at the nurses' stations. Sneakers squeak on linoleum; every sound is amplified during the night, and you hear sounds you never notice during the day. Your watch ticks loudly, your stomach growls, the nurse at the desk a little ways down the hall shifts in her squeaky chair as she tries to find a comfortable position. Your patient's ventilator hums, purrs, and thumps a comfortingly metronomic forced respiration.

Nurses smelling strongly of coffee and fabric softener pass by, their cotton-swaddled thighs announcing their arrivals and departures with a coarse *swish-swish*; you don't need to look up or turn around to know who's who. An infant cries, a teenager moans, and you can hear the hushed voices of pediatric specialists as they confer over the respiratory failure in room seven.

Charts land with a muffled thud on desktops. Pens scratch about the body's inner workings, its failures. The pages turn without giving a thought to the human being they represent.

It is only midnight, and you are already struggling to stay awake. You have another seven hours to go. Hourly checks begin now. It is dark in the room and hard to see, and you use a flashlight to avoid waking your patients with the sudden shock of bright overhead lights. Whisper your name, explain your mission, and flash your penlight into unresponsive pupils. Feel for pulses: bounding, thready, absent. Examine abdomens: soft, distended, hard, rigid. Listen to lungs: coarse, bubbling, raspy. Inspect urine and tubing. Inspect the machines that control, monitor, and report every breath, heartbeat, movement, and drop of intravenous solutions.

Parents sleep curled together on tiny cots, huddled under thin white blankets. Parents wake and hover at bedsides, gently touching their child's hair, hands, and sheets. Some just stand, wringing their hands or tucking them into pockets, their eyes welling with tears, their lips twisting against sorrow, despair, and helplessness. You can smell their grief: sharp, tangy, and sweaty, like the insides of sneakers no longer new but not yet old. If you breathe too deeply, the smell here is overwhelming—besides the despair, there are also the odors of antiseptics, bleached linens, floor cleaner, metal instruments, blood, urine, feces, and death. You wonder why you come here, night after night.

Go back to your cubicle, nestled between two patients' rooms, far enough away to safely disconnect from their sorrow, yet not so far that you won't hear a cough, an alarm, or a soft voice calling for Mommy. You write your findings in little boxes ordered conveniently by hour and body system. Hundreds of little boxes the size of your pinky fingernail allow no room for words, only codes: A for alert, B for semiconscious, C for comatose. There are no codes for fearful or crying, but there are codes for the color of urine, the numbers and locations of inserted tubes and needles, the settings on the machines, the fluids infusing into tiny veins. Pain is assigned a scale from one to ten, but there is no number for pain beyond ten, and you rarely see a one. There is no box where you can write "the pain killers don't work anymore" or "Dad is having trouble coping" or "she was too drugged to watch her favorite TV show before bed."

You check them again at one in the morning, and again at two, three, and four. At four o'clock, you draw blood, which you hope will be the most interesting and difficult part of your night, though this is rarely the case. With a flashlight, you examine tiny hands, arms, feet, and legs with even tinier veins that seem to run and hide the minute a needle appears. The child watches, patiently accepting the impending torture, allowing you to slide a needle in and adjust the position left and right, down and up, as you try to pierce the sneaky vein. They bite their lower lips, trying to be strong, little victims of medical science's constant need to analyze and fill more boxes. When you can't get it, you call another nurse who examines the child's limbs with a flashlight, illuminating the veins from below. She swabs the area with alcohol, inserts another needle, and twists it from side to side, up and down, sliding it this way and that without removing it from beneath the skin. Sometimes she is lucky, or sometimes a third or fourth nurse must be called. When the trauma is over, we leave the room, sit at our desks, and fill in the little boxes. We grab coffee from the break room. We chat with each other about our kids' soccer games, the tomatoes growing in the garden, our lovers, husbands, and neighbors, but never our patients.

Alarms sound all night from IV pumps, oxygen monitors, and feeding tubes, but there is one alarm that still makes you jump and sends chills down your spine. When that one sounds, it's rarely due to a malfunction or loose wires, though you always hope that's the case. Everyone on the unit comes running. People from other units too. One person pushes a large metal cart, its drawers stuffed full of medical supplies, while another carries a chart (with more little boxes) and another a defibrillator. People shout orders—"Give me one milligram of atropine!"—and needles plunge into the IV port; a nurse kneeling on the bed compresses a tiny chest, sheets puffing out around her from the force of her downward thrusts, as another nurse forces air into the patient's lungs with a resuscitation bag. Others have gathered around the bed and pushed the parents out of the room. The physician calls out, "All clear?" and everyone's hands go up into the air like we're about to cheer.

The defibrillator emits a long, high-pitched beep. We all wait to hear the heart monitor call out a steady rhythm. It usually doesn't, and the frantic scene is repeated in its entirety for another twenty minutes or more, or until the heart beats again. Sometimes it works. A lot of times it doesn't. A hush falls over everyone when the doctor announces, "I'm calling it." No one makes eye contact as you bustle about picking up paper scraps, the empty bottles of injected drugs, the fallen bed linens. The child is covered to the neck with a clean sheet, and there is a screeching, desperate, and animal-like wail in the hallway as the mom and dad realize their baby is gone. Other parents, clenching their own fists and thanking God it wasn't their child, poke their heads from their children's rooms and look on with sympathy and fear at the now-childless couple. Nurses pat the grief-stricken parents on their shoulders and return to their desks to fill out the little boxes. One nurse will stop to take them by the hand, lead them to the body, and give them time to be alone with their child.

Survivors are woken at 5:00 a.m. Baths are given, dressings changed. Residents come in and perform exams in preparation for 7:00 a.m. rounds with their superiors. Linens are changed. Awakened parents head out for coffee, breakfast, and respite. Back at your desk to again fill in the little boxes; write small notes in the chart about anything that doesn't fit inside them. (You are cautioned to write only objective findings. Grief, sorrow, and helplessness are not objective—stick to colors, numbers, and other measurable things that don't have a box.)

The next shift of box fillers begins to arrive, and you chat with them about your family, your tomatoes, your husband. You discuss the little boxes as you stand in the doorway of your patient's room, commenting on urine color, the infusing solutions, the drugs you injected, the surgery he will be taken to, just had, or was too sick to have.

You envelop yourself in your coat, pull it tightly around you, and bury your hands deep in its pockets as you walk to your car, head down. You drive home as the sun rises and climb into bed, thankful for the cocoon of soft sheets, pillows, and quiet; your neighbor, lover, or husband heads to work. The tomatoes are busy ripening in the garden, and the children are off at school, talking about the next big soccer game. Oblivious to the drama that occurred on the night shift, the day unfolds while you sleep.

DENISE ELLIOTT *is a registered nurse currently working in palliative care; she has spent the past twenty-four years working in both pediatric and adult nursing. She has two grown children and resides in Southern California.*

A LONG NIGHT'S JOURNEY INTO DAY

Theresa Brown

A clinical nurse has been advocating for a patient who agrees to accept a risky treatment—but who refuses any lifesaving measures in the event of complications. Now, she is tasked with administering the drug that could end her patient's life.

Rose, a mother in her forties with young kids, had gotten an allogeneic stem cell transplant—an allo—with the hope it would cure her cancer. In and out of the hospital for several months afterward, she dealt with a lot of bad side effects; unremitting bloody and black diarrhea was the reason for her most recent admission, and the docs now wanted to try a last-ditch drug that might help her. It could also make her so sick that she'd need intensive care to save her life.

And she was refusing to go to the ICU.

Her nurse that day, Anne, was a young woman with a strikingly beautiful face and the courage to speak her mind. The wisdom and bravery she displayed in this situation were impressive, considering her age.

"She doesn't want it," she insisted to anyone who would listen. "She doesn't want to go to the ICU."

The medical staff felt differently. To give such a potentially toxic drug to a patient, they argued, imposed the ethical obligation to save her from the drug's possibly lethal effects. Rose, however, did not want to be saved.

I first met Rose during one of the many admissions that followed her allo. Or maybe that was when she first really caught my attention. She'd developed a rash that turned her face purple. This can happen as a result of graft-versus-host disease, a side effect of allogeneic transplants, but it's nonetheless surreal to see a human patient so resemble a blueberry. I was taking over her care from the dayshift nurse during the midday shift change.

She had horrible diarrhea that time, too, and was using the portable commode we'd set up in her room when I heard her moan and saw her collapse in on herself. The dayshift nurse and I couldn't rouse her. Worried she'd had a seizure, or that something equally bad had happened, we called in a rapid response team, and the room quickly filled with people. Other nurses from the oncology floor, ICU nurses, a physician who specialized in intensive care patients (called an intensivist), and a respiratory therapist all came in while the poor woman sat on the toilet. Her husband, Toby, tried to use his body to shield her, protecting her dignity while inadvertently obstructing the medical care she needed.

The intensivist let out a small sigh and asked if we could move Rose onto the bed. She weighed very little. But then she was once again alert. I helped her to stand and shuffle back to her bed to lie down. I looked down at the bucket in the bedside commode, full of black liquid that looked like nothing that should, or even could, come from a human gastrointestinal tract.

If I'd been in her position, I would have worried that one could actually die of embarrassment. Once Rose returned from wherever she briefly went while we couldn't revive her, she was nonetheless calm and helpful, answering questions clearly, neither minimizing nor overdramatizing what had happened.

She hadn't seized. Her blood pressure was through the roof, but that wasn't surprising, considering the stress she probably felt at that moment. Her skin was purple, and something was very obviously wrong with her gut, but nothing was so acutely wrong that it required a code team to pile into her room as she went to the bathroom. And she certainly did not need to be cared for in the ICU.

Everyone else left, and the dayshift nurse and I explained why we'd called in the code team. "There are times when we need more help," we said. "Now you know that if there's a real crisis, we have all these people ready to step in."

• • •

In time, Rose's skin cleared, her GI system returned to normal, more or less, and she went home. Anytime a long-term patient leaves the hospital, it's a happy day for her and the staff; for me, Rose's returning home felt especially significant. She and I were roughly the same age, our children were the same ages, and we both had PhDs that we weren't using in our present lives: I had gone into nursing; she was home with her children. She'd had such a rough ride posttransplant, and her young kids, her devoted husband, and her own graciousness and focus all made Rose a patient whose well-being I became personally invested in.

In an allogeneic transplant, cancer patients receive intravenous infusions of someone else's hematopoietic (blood-making) stem cells, which include the cells that had contributed to the donor's immune system. The donated cells are the graft, the patient, the host. Unfortunately, the graft cells can attack the patient. This is graft-versus-host disease, or GVHD, and it's what happened when Rose's skin turned blue. The skin and digestive system problems that Rose developed after her transplant had been symptoms of acute disease. Her many subsequent readmissions to the hospital, also due to skin and gut problems, suggested the more chronic form of GVHD. The severity of the disease varies, but at its most aggressive, it can kill as surely as cancer.

In the first few months after her transplant, Rose developed a rash unlike the one that had turned her face purple, a red rash that spread all over her body. Her skin began to slough off, giving her the appearance of a burn victim. Our doctors thought a complicated procedure called photopheresis might help, so Rose started going by ambulance to a different hospital with a photopheresis machine. The process took four hours, and when she returned to the hospital, her bedside nurse would apply medicated lotion to her skin and wrap it in Saran Wrap, trying to keep inside whatever moisture remained.

I was never her nurse during this time, but I saw what she went through— the uncomfortable ambulance rides, the slow and painful wrapping of her skin. She displayed incredible fortitude, commenting gently when something hurt, putting up with the annoying trips to the other hospital. On the floor, she walked in the hall as often as she could, dutifully performing the strengthening exercises detailed by signs posted at intervals along the walls: Stand on one leg, then the other. Do push-ups off the wall.

"What choice do I have?" she would say when I noted how hard she was working to stay strong.

She would get better, go home, and invariably return to the hospital. Every time she left, we sighed with relief, crossed our fingers, wished her never back. Whenever she returned, I got a hollow feeling in my stomach. She was such a wonderful person, and her illness trajectory seemed so unfair. The resemblances between her life and mine left me constantly fearful for her husband and children, and for my own.

Things never went well for Rose for long. Too soon, she came back to the hospital with terrible diarrhea, agreeing to treatment with another powerful drug but refusing a transfer to the ICU.

She wasn't my patient, but Anne wanted some help speaking for Rose, and I butted in. I was at the nurse's station when the situation unfolded. It was the middle of the afternoon, and I'd just come in for evening shift, from three in the afternoon to eleven at night. Both Rose's doctor and her husband wanted her to take the drug. And she was willing. But she didn't want to go to intensive care, be put on a ventilator, and be loaded up with lines and tubes. She had physically suffered so much already; ICU was a line she refused to cross.

The clinical pharmacist on her case, David, had a surprising and wry sense of humor. On that day, though, he was thoroughly serious, arguing that it was unethical to give Rose a potentially toxic drug and then stand by to watch as it killed her. If, through our care, we created a life-threatening situation for Rose, he maintained, then we needed to do everything we could to reverse the dangerous effects of our treatment.

His reasoning was sound, his logic flawless—the patient simply disagreed. She would take the drug but would go no further to save her own life.

"People are complicated," I told him when he said that Rose's decision made no sense. It made sense to Anne and me. Perhaps, being women, we more instinctively understood the necessity of compromise in such a situation. She would take the drug for the men in her life—and, by extension, for her children—but she refused to abandon her autonomy over her own body. Anne and I had also seen the physical toll of her treatments, with not much good health to show for it.

We convinced the medical team that we would administer the drug but would refrain from calling a code or initiating Rose's transfer to the ICU in the event of a bad reaction. To cover ourselves legally, we clearly indicated these choices on the required Code Status form and carefully documented Rose's decision. The treatment would start that evening, after Anne finished her shift. The nurse in charge had just asked me to work for sixteen hours, which meant I would stay overnight until seven thirty the next morning. I agreed, and she then told me I would be Rose's nurse for the rest of the shift.

So began the longest night of my life. The drug would drip in over the course of several hours, and I would be taking vital signs often. Toby planned to stay the night. I doubted he would sleep at all.

If Rose crashed and we couldn't save her on the floor, she would die. Toby had agreed to this plan, her wish. It had all made sense when Anne and I argued on her behalf; but now that I was charged with carrying out Rose's wishes, I wasn't sure how I would manage.

Fortunately, one can always fall back on routine. I gave Rose the premedications she needed before the IV infusion started. I then waited for pharmacy to deliver the drug, double-checked the dose in the IV bag against the written order, and started the infusion. There was no drama in any of these tasks. I was giving meds and hooking up an IV, both of which I'd done hundreds of times.

The drug dripped in—nothing happened. Because the situation with Rose could turn critical at any moment, the charge nurse had assigned me only three patients. My other two were cakewalks, thank goodness, who needed little from me.

Rose's blood pressure was a little off during the first few hours as the drug infused. Every time I took her vital signs, Toby insisted on hearing the numbers himself, and I would read off her heart rate, oxygen level, blood pressure, respiratory rate, and temperature. He would then look at me, trying to read my reaction. I strove to project a calm watchfulness; I'm not sure I succeeded. I could honestly reassure him, though, that she was stable. Her oxygen needs weren't increasing, and her heart rate wasn't going crazy. Her blood pressure was a little funky but nowhere near dangerous.

Rose mostly slept, and when she woke up, it was because I was clumsy taking her vitals or because she had more diarrhea, but not because she was worried or suffering.

Regardless of her calm, every set of vitals felt like an ordeal. The blood pressure cuff was attached to a dial on the wall by a long, curled cord that twisted and pulled awkwardly whenever I used it. Pulling the cuff toward Rose, I would invariably slide the cord across her face or drag it along the top of her head. Then I'd wrap the blood pressure cuff around her wasted upper arm, gently put the bell of the stethoscope under the edge of the cuff, and pump up the bulb that registered her pressure. The pulse oximeter—which I'd attached to a finger on her opposite hand—registered her oxygen saturation and heart rate while I released the air in the bulb and listened for her pressure. I'd then take the cuff off her arm, unclip the pulse ox from her finger, and stick an aural thermometer in her ear.

It felt like a dumb show. It was dark outside, and the dim light over Rose's sink was the only light in the room. I did my work with the cuff and the pulse ox monitor, trying to appear impassive while Toby watched me, apprehensive. I whispered the numbers to him. Rose did her best to sleep. It took about five minutes to take her vitals, and we did the whole thing all over again every thirty minutes.

At around two in the morning, I realized that Rose was going to be OK. If someone's body will react to the drug, it usually happens at the beginning of the infusion. She'd been mostly stable, even at the start. The change I'd noticed in her blood pressure, earlier, had resolved itself over the past few hours.

I told Toby that she would be all right and suggested he try to sleep. He couldn't. I'm sure he was tired, but how could any man sleep through the night when his wife, partly as a result of her own choices, might have died? If we had gotten to that point, he would have surely wanted a chance to say good-bye. He was a kind man, friendly, generous. But that night—all night—he projected a tense wariness that wore on me. He had been ready for his wife to die, and now she would live. I don't know anyone who could adjust easily to such a change, and he seemed stuck. He'd been prepared for the worst, but now a small bit of hope quietly entered the room. Could he believe in it?

I confess that I was not so diligent with my vital signs over the next three hours. I went in only every hour and disconnected the empty drug bag at around five in the morning. Rose slept, Toby also. His vigil was over.

In Eugene O'Neill's play *A Long Day's Journey into Night*, the members of an emotionally mistrustful family try, and fail, to find a way to care for each other. The father, formerly a famous actor, is a self-absorbed skinflint, and the mother is a morphine addict. The younger son has tuberculosis, the older a lifetime of resentment. They feel attached to one another, but caught up as they are in their own preoccupations and needs, their attachments are ambivalent, hurtful. By the end of the play, night has fallen, the male characters are alienated from each other, and the mother is so doped up that she's lost touch with reality.

My night with Rose and Toby was a reversal of that narrative trajectory. We had feared that the night would bring about the ultimate fracturing of their family—the death of a much-loved wife and mother—but she survived, and her husband stayed with her to loyally offer his support throughout the night. Day and light would come for them both.

Before I left for home that morning, I went to see Rose one last time. She woke when I came into the room, and the look on her face was devastating. She was—disappointed. I saw it: the tightening around her eyes, the quick and sad downturn at the corners of her mouth. It was a brief, unguarded moment before she recovered her usual equanimity, but it was enough for me to learn something unexpected: she was sorry she hadn't died. The look on her face suggested—to me, at least—that she wanted the drug to have killed her.

Toby woke up at that moment, so I couldn't ask Rose how she felt about having made it through the night. Besides, a new day was starting: the first flickers of dawn would soon light up the world outside the windows; a new nurse would come in to take over for me; the doctors would begin to assess whether the drug had done any good.

In the end, it didn't. Rose got the drug a few more times, during daylight and with much less drama, and although it didn't kill her, neither did it save her. A few weeks after that long night—after more drugs, more days of horrible diarrhea, and at the end, more pain—she died.

The morning after that first dose, dazed with exhaustion and the emotional strain of my shift, I left work wondering how I would ever recover professionally from such an ordeal. I'd given a patient a drug that could have killed her, and I would have watched her die without sounding an alarm or calling in more help, knowing that I was doing my job well. Before that night with Rose, I hadn't understood that being a good nurse might entail such a friendly intimacy with death.

Feeling more tired than I'd ever felt after work, I walked outside through the sliding glass doors leading to the small alley that separated the parking garage from the hospital. I usually experienced this passage as a sort of limbo: a seven-foot-long stretch of asphalt that got me to where I parked, a portal where tired nurses left as fresh ones entered. On that morning, though, I felt a breeze on my face as I stepped through the double doors and saw the day's first light, and it hit me: *I'm alive.*

THERESA BROWN, BSN, RN, OCN, *is a clinical nurse and sole contributor to the* New York Times *opinion column Bedside. She is the author of* Critical Care: A New Nurse Faces Death, Life, and Everything in Between, *a memoir of her first year in nursing.* Critical Care *has been adopted as a textbook by many schools of nursing, and she lectures nationally on issues related to nursing and healthcare.*

DON'T EVER FORGET ME

Christopher Lance Coleman

A professor of nursing remembers being a student at the onset of the AIDS epidemic in the 1980s, when treatments were nearly nonexistent and funeral homes refused to pick up those who died from the disease. Today he worries that the harsh realities of the disease are being forgotten.

B ack then, there was no hope for anybody.

There was no hope for the woman behind the hospital door on which a sign was posted: Patient Has AIDS. Do Not Enter. There was no hope for the man with Kaposi's sarcoma, whose eyes turned black as he bled out. There was no hope for the couple who came to hospice together and died within weeks of one another.

It was the advent of AIDS, the 1980s, and I was a nursing student. Nursing students weren't allowed to take care of patients with AIDS, then, which I thought strange. Why couldn't we? Nurses take care of everybody. One evening I was at the nurses' station and could hear a patient crying in her room, the room behind the door with the warning sign. I walked in. Her dinner was sitting on her bedside tray. Her fork was on the floor. I asked her what was the matter.

"I dropped my fork," she said.

"Have you had anything to eat today?"

"I can't. I can't lift my hand up." She was so sick, so emaciated and weak. I took her food out, warmed it in the microwave, and fed her.

The hospital wanted nurses treating AIDS patients to wear gowns that covered bodies and faces. It looked as if we were approaching a biohazard, and I refused to put it on. I had read enough to know that this disease was transmitted through bodily fluids and required only gloves and universal precautions. Nevertheless, I was reprimanded by the nurses and my instructor for being an ungowned student in the room of a patient with AIDS.

I promised myself that I would never let this happen to another human being. A patient had been sitting there, hungry, and no one had fed her. I was determined to work with folks with AIDS.

That promise led to my career in HIV/AIDS hospice care and my research in HIV/AIDS prevention. We are now seeing people with HIV/AIDS live for decades—long enough to add another layer to the US healthcare crisis introduced by the aging baby boomers. Sadly, today's young people with AIDS seem not to think much of it; they don't remember those who wasted and died from the disease.

In the '80s, it was called GRID: gay-related immune deficiency syndrome. That's what appeared in the newspapers, and that's what was on the TV news. It was a scary time. The doctors didn't know what it was, and there were all kinds of conspiracy theories: the government was trying to kill people, or the disease was being brought from Africa.

I very clearly remember hearing from my ministers in church that the disease wouldn't touch African Americans, that we were safe because we were moral, and that this was a disease of gay, white men. I heard that over and over. I had looked around and felt comforted that it wasn't going to strike anybody I knew. But I also remember asking myself, *What's going to happen when the disease moves beyond gay, white males?*

A Dignified Death

It was a bad time for anybody who had AIDS or was HIV positive. You would hear the term *sick*, as in "so-and-so is sick." People were dying. There was no treatment.

I was working in Oregon as a nurse and was connected with a Quaker organization that supported the notion of dignified deaths for men with

HIV and AIDS. It was not even considered, at the time, whether someone with AIDS deserved to die with dignity. Besides, nobody expected young people to die, though they were dying in large numbers.

The Quakers purchased an old nursing home and, in the face of the neighborhood's homophobia, we created a safe haven inside it. We called it Our House. It was the first AIDS hospice in the state. I became the director and was initially the only RN, the only one licensed to give the Schedule II drugs that would help our men with the dying process.

There was no medical regimen to help them die more peacefully. If somebody had cancer, you knew what medications to give as that person got closer to death. No one yet believed that AIDS patients had pain, and we had to fight to get our residents pain medication.

We would not let anyone die without dignity. Whenever someone died, we held a ceremony in our recreation room, and all available staff and able residents came to share their stories about that person. Most of the time, we honored the person's memory with a symbolic activity—we planted a tree in our outdoor garden, lit a candle, found a way to wish him well on his journey.

When our men first started to die, we couldn't get the funeral homes to pick them up, and we sometimes had to call an ambulance to take them. One funeral home sent their staff outfitted in full biohazard suits. One of the residents hurried over to me and took me by the hand. "Do not let me go out of here like that." I didn't let anyone go out like that again. We had to educate funeral homes about AIDS. We started a ritual where we would lay a quilt on our deceased men and walk their bodies out to the hearse. Everybody got to see them go out. It was like our flag of tribute to the person's life.

We honored their lives. We honored their deaths. But we wouldn't say good-bye: we would always say, "Good journey." It took the fear from many of our residents. When our people were ready to die, they would say, "I'm ready to take my journey. I'm ready to go." It helped the staff to get in touch with the reality of death too. It was such a challenging time.

• • •

The Short Season

Our friends started to come into the hospice for care, but we didn't recognize them. They would look at me and ask, "Don't you know who I am?" and I would reply, "No, I don't recognize you." The virus had so thoroughly changed their appearances. It was incredibly hard on the guys, so young and vital just four or five months before, who had been out partying, having a good time, living their lives with their friends. Some would never leave the residence because they didn't want to be seen. These were young people with a horrible disease that was killing off their bodies, but their youthful souls, full of energy, were so strong; they wanted to live.

We worked hard to educate these young men that it was OK to die; some people will live for a short season, some people will live for a longer season, we would say, and nobody knows when his season will end. When they understood this, they took a perspective that seemed to say, *I have AIDS, and I'm going to live my life the best I can in my final days, and then I'm going to die.* It struck me that when someone was ready to go, he went fast.

We on the staff would prepare ourselves for our patients who were likely to die. There's a term for this: *nurse's intuition.* After you've seen a phenomenon occur often enough, you begin to know when it is coming again. I often knew who would die next, and I would immediately start preparing that person for death.

Jon was our first Native American patient. He had internalized Kaposi's sarcoma, which typically appears on the skin as purple spots. Additionally, the disease had disseminated throughout his body and had gone to all his organs. We knew it was likely that he would bleed out, and he did. It was horrible. His eyes turned black; blood started to emanate from every orifice. He drowned in his blood. Moments earlier, he had been alert and awake—it happened so quickly. It was part of his culture to believe he was curable, and Jon's last words to me were, "Don't let me die." The words haunted me for a long time. I held his hand and told him, "It's OK, it's OK. Take your journey."

Men like Jon made me appreciate the dying process. It is work. I had seen death before, but those deaths were heart attacks or cardiac arrests; they were patients who died in the ER or were brought in already dead. But watching a young person struggle with death—that was something for which I was unprepared.

We found that some of our residents were having hard times with the dying process because they hadn't made peace with people in their lives. In most of these cases, their families had turned their backs on them. We felt it was especially important for them to make peace with their mothers, who became extremely crucial components of our care. They were the most willing to visit their sons. I held the hands of many mothers who came to the hospice.

We created a home setting for our men at Our House. Volunteers prepared homecooked meals, and the staff was expected to join in the nightly sit-down dinner with the residents. The healthier residents had chores. We had a garden and ran field trips. We also allowed our residents to bring furnishings from their homes so they could surround themselves with a semblance of the lives they'd lived before they got sick. This was unheard of, at the time. Although we weren't officially allowed to have pets, we welcomed therapy animals. And we did surreptitiously permit a pet dog or two that would curl up on the beds.

Professionally and personally, I have lost a lot of people to AIDS—colleagues, friends, people who I was shocked to learn had it, people who didn't tell me they had it. I remember when our first heterosexual couple came in; both of them were absolutely beautiful. It was the first time we had a female staying at Our House. Females have all kinds of different symptomatology and conditions with HIV/AIDS, and the medication we had at the time did almost nothing for her. He died, and she died soon after.

This field invited me into a world that I would have otherwise avoided completely. My heart and soul was in it, and it was the right thing to do. Any challenges I experienced were nothing compared to what these men had gone through.

My friends buried and resurrected me I don't know how many times. People created all kinds of stories about you, back then: they thought that

I had died of AIDS somewhere. There was a stigma to the work I was doing. But I eventually got to a point where I wasn't afraid to say, when someone asked what I did, "I work with persons who are dying of AIDS."

No Way to Live, No Way to Die

Thirty years later, we still don't have a cure. We have great treatments that keep people alive longer, and this is terrific, but there is a price we all pay for longer lives. Our government is not prepared for the cohort of people with AIDS who are going to retire and enter the healthcare system, and many of whom will receive Medicare or Medicaid benefits.

People are still dying from AIDS, of course, but it's not like it was. Today people with HIV/AIDS also die from causes like old age, which is an incredible development I never thought I'd see in my lifetime. If somebody had told me, back then, that people with HIV/AIDS would someday live to fifty, sixty, or seventy years of age, I would have looked at that person and laughed. That wasn't what we saw. People were lucky if they lived to be thirty-five years old.

I truly fear for the young people who are getting infected, who presume that it's not so bad and that everything will be fine for them. Young people have no clue what HIV/AIDS can do to their bodies or what the long-term effects of the drug treatments can entail.

At the same time, very few people are going into infectious disease care. Who will take care of these new patients? We no longer have wards dedicated to AIDS, and we have very few nurses who know how care for an AIDS patient.

Considering the ways in which the healthcare system is being cut back, I wonder what will be left for the young people who are infected now. What will be there for them when they're old? I see a lack of vigilance, a lack of concern. As we approach the thirty-year anniversary of HIV/AIDS, we need to put this issue back on the front page of the paper.

Having AIDS is no way to live. The now-dead guys I had cared for, if they were alive today, would tell young people to protect themselves; they would tell them it's no cakewalk.

At Our House, the guys would often say, "Don't forget me." "I won't forget you," I would promise. I can remember every single one of their faces. We cannot forget them, and we cannot forget AIDS.

CHRISTOPHER LANCE COLEMAN, PHD, *is the Fagin Term Associate Professor of Nursing and Multicultural Diversity and is codirector of the Center for Health Equity Research at the University of Pennsylvania School of Nursing. He has published research articles and book chapters, served on numerous boards, and received both federal and intramural funding for AIDS research. His book,* Dangerous Intimacy: Ten African American Men with HIV, *is the result of his work with seropositive men.*

HEART LESSONS

Diane Kraynak

The maternity ward is usually a joyful place, but it has its share of tragedy, too. A NICU nurse remembers her attempts to document the brief life of an infant who would never leave the hospital.

The heart is not my favorite organ. It seems complicated. Four chambers, an aorta, and a few valves. Pressure drives blood in, pressure forces blood out. I shouldn't be intimidated by a ten-ounce muscled pump, but I am.

I remember trying to stay awake during the cardiovascular session of a two-day review class for pediatric nurse practitioners (PNPs). The instructor, Bernie, described the anatomy and the different types of heart failure in simple and elegant detail. But it was late in the morning of the second day, and my brain was cooked. I passed my PNP exam, which only had a few heart questions, but I continued to work as a newborn intensive care unit nurse. I was gaining experience before I had to be the nurse practitioner, the one who made the decisions. Despite the review, despite Bernie, despite passing, I still thought hearts were complicated. I did not like them.

My own heart was fragile right then, though not physically. That summer's love interest, Dan, had kicked me to the curb at the end of August. It still smarted. My aching heart preoccupied me as I sped down I-64 to work the NICU day shift. I was going to be in Dan's town the following day for a college football game. *Would I run into him?*

Inside the massive concrete parking deck, I grabbed my lunch, coffee, and purse. The car's clock said 6:59. Eight minutes to punch in. Despite Dan, despite my melancholy, it was going to be a good day.

I glanced at the assignment sheet, saw my name written in a bed space, and ambled over toward the real bed in the unit. A silver-haired nurse approached, my friend Sue Birch. Sue, who worked nights, was a warm, motherly figure who supplied the unit with jumbo packs of Twizzlers and donned kooky glasses to make us laugh when tensions rose. She was too young to be my mother and too old to be my sister. She was someone in between, and with my own family an hour away, I gravitated to her.

"Birch," I said. "What's going on?"

"Hi, honey." She dug in her scrubs pocket for lipstick.

"Where's my baby?" I said, as she painted her lips.

"This little one is your sole assignment." She handed me my Kardex, the printed sheet that organized the patient's vital signs, laboratory values, fluid balances, and medications in perfect Arial ten. I folded it lengthwise and got ready to take notes.

"Go," I said.

She began. "This is Lamonica, a thirty-eight-weeker, born last night via C-section. Left hypoplastic heart. The echo's getting progressively worse. They knew about the heart condition before birth, but it's worse than they thought. She's too sick to cath, and surgery is now out of the question. Palliative care only."

I wrote furiously on the baby's Kardex, covering the page, trying to capture all the information.

"Anyway," Sue continued, "we just turned off her IV fluids and stopped feeds. She was extubated an hour ago. Mom's upstairs, but she's coming down after report. They saw the baby for a few minutes after the delivery, but that was it. Parents not married. I hear they're real nice. There's another family in the Quiet Room. The on-call room is empty, if the family wants to go in there."

I let out a long breath and looked at Sue. "I hate hearts."

"I'm sorry, honey."

"That's OK."

"We thought you'd be the best to take her."

"Lucky me."

"We have so many new grads . . ."

"Scary to think I'm the experienced one."

"Why don't you come over tonight? We're marinating something."

"Let's see how today goes."

"All right," she said. She handed me a paper towel. Inside was a Twizzler. I laughed.

"Sleep tight," I said to her back as she left.

I'd been in the NICU for a year and a half. Despite the usual and expected infant mortality there, I hadn't had much experience with death. Lamonica was my second baby to die, but my first baby for whom we turned off life support.

I peered into her warming table. At a glance, you wouldn't know she was dying, but if you got closer, you knew something wasn't right. Her heart condition made her cocoa skin bluish. The worn white blanket and overhead fluorescents turned her bluer still. Her eyes were closed. She was breathing heavily.

My mind went back to that PNP review class. Hypoplastic heart. Underdevelopment of left ventricle, mitral valve, aortic valve, and ascending aortic arch. The left side couldn't do its job, so the right side had to work for both. But the right side couldn't sustain both sides for long—not without surgical intervention.

I took off her hat and rubbed my hand over her head. Her black hair was soft; her tender fontanel pulsed under my fingers.

"Hey, sweet girl," I said, stroking her cheeks.

Her eyes opened. Onyx orbs observed me, reflecting the overhead lights in two white spots.

Light reflex, good.

She gulped air. *Mucous membranes moist, cyanotic.*

I gently placed my stethoscope on her chest. She breathed rapidly. *Lung sound clear and equal bilaterally.* Though I could hear the heart murmur from her lungs, I also had to listen to her heart. It told the story.

Whoosh, whoosh, whoosh instead of *lub-dub, lub-dub, lub-dub.*

I slid the stethoscope down her soft belly. Her umbilical cord rose like a purple stalk above her diaper, drying and dying. *Abdomen soft, nontender; liver and spleen normal size.*

I opened her diaper. *Normal female. Tanner I. Full range of motion. Two plus edema on her extremities. Feet cool to touch. Blood pressure 60/30.* Shit.

The overhead page blasted: "Nurse taking care of Baby Lamonica, line one. Nurse taking care of Baby Lamonica, line one."

"This is Diane," I said.

It was the maternity ward, asking if Mom and the family could come down.

"Yes. Send them down."

A grave group shuffled up to Lamonica's warming table. "I'm Diane. I'm taking care of her today," I said. "Mom?" I asked, raising my eyebrows to the woman hunched in a wheelchair. She was wearing a green hospital gown. Her hair was matted, her face ashen. She nodded.

"You're Dad?" I said to the man next to her.

"Levon," he said, touching his collar. "This is Leslie," pointing to Mom. "Grandma, Grandma, Grandpa," he said, introducing the rest of the group.

We nodded at one another, grim faced but polite.

"We can go to the on-call room. It's private and a little more comfortable," I said. Mom nodded.

"Do you want to carry her?" I asked.

"You can," Mom said.

I picked her up. Lamonica was soft and cuddly. She stirred against me. I rarely held an infant; we didn't hold babies in the NICU. We couldn't. These babies slumbered in incubators or warming tables, fighting illnesses and catching up to their expected birth dates. Something about babies—their size and their sleepiness—made it seem like all was well with the world. But all was not right in Lamonica's world. She had only half a heart. And nothing was right in her family's world. They followed me into the on-call room.

I opened the door and cringed. Fatigue, sweat, and old food infused the saggy, dingy cushions on the clunky wooden furniture. Black scuffs marked the gray-white walls.

I handed Lamonica to Mom and leaned against the wall to stay out of the way. Mom brought her face down to her daughter's and rubbed noses. Dad stooped over them. Lamonica blinked at her parents.

They passed her around and took turns cooing, touching, and stroking her. Someone finally passed her to Dad. He grabbed her awkwardly.

"Cradle her, Levon," one of the grandmothers said.

Dad shifted her up on his arm, his eyes wide, his lips tight.

"That's better," the grandmother said.

The room hushed. The family wept. We waited. Lamonica was my only assignment, so I waited with them.

My mind wouldn't settle down. Nothing in nursing school had prepared me for this. I surveyed the scene and tried to corral my thoughts. *Am I really supposed to sit here? Should I be talking to them?*

It was six weeks since I'd seen Dan. *Would he be at the game tomorrow? Would I run into him?*

I wriggled my toes in my tennis shoes and shifted against the wall. *I could go to Sue's for dinner. Sue didn't really tell me how this works. Do I hover? Do I leave them?* Mom was humming to Lamonica. My mind hummed with her.

"I'll come back to check on you," I said.

"OK," said Mom.

When I came back, Lamonica was still alive and in her father's arms. Mom was in pain. She wanted to go and get Percocet.

"Sure. I'll call your nurse." They returned their daughter to me. Sharon, the nurse manager, lingered nearby in case I needed help. She took Lamonica from me so I could help Mom to the elevators where her nurse, Trina, was waiting for us. Mom slid further down in her wheelchair, collapsing in on herself.

"Hey, Diane," Trina said.

"Hey." We had been nursing school classmates.

"I'll bring her right back."

"We'll be here."

Trina was sympathetic. Lamonica's plight reached into the maternity ward as well. I would soon lose my patient, but Mom, not ready to go home, would still be in Trina's care.

Back in the unit, Lamonica cuddled in Sharon's arms. As I approached, however, Lamonica turned blue. Sharon started vigorous rubs on Lamonica's back and flicked her feet to stimulate her. I grabbed the oxygen, and we inched our way over to Lamonica's warming table. Sharon and I looked at each other, sharing the same thought: this baby was not going to die without her mother.

Here, too, were things not taught in any nursing class: the unspoken communication, invisible and unacknowledged; the silent gestures that showed what was needed, and which we understood intuitively; the help and care that made a tragic situation less unbearable.

Jamie, another nurse in the unit, saw what we were doing and came over. Her chin came up and her spine straightened with immediate understanding.

"Jamie? Can you call Eight and get Mom back here?" I said. Sharon and I had laid Lamonica in her warming table. I took the oxygen from Lamonica's mouth, keeping one eye on the monitor, one eye on her. Her heart rate was fast but better, and she was less blue. Sharon and I had bought her more time, but not much.

"No problem," Jamie said, her hand already on the phone.

"Diane, line one. Diane, line one," blared the overhead page.

"Take it," Sharon said. "I've got her."

"This is Diane."

"Hey. It's Karen. Can you be ready around nine tomorrow? The game starts—"

I interrupted. "My baby's dying. Can I call you later?"

"Oh my God."

"I'll call you later."

I returned my attention to Lamonica. Sharon had bundled her up again. She passed her to me. "You got her?"

"Yeah, I'm good."

"Need anything?" Jamie asked. She had been a classmate also.

I turned to Jamie. "No. I just want to keep her alive until Mom gets back."

"Why did she leave?"

"Percocet."

"Maybe she didn't want to be around."

I stopped bouncing and patting Lamonica. I exhaled and looked at Jamie. I hadn't thought of that. Lamonica and I paced our corner. She was less blue, but her breathing was a slow, rhythmic wheeze. I glanced around the unit at all the other nurses busy with their babies. In the clamor of monitors, vents, phones, and beeps, all I heard was Lamonica.

Jamie leaned over and caressed her face.

"She's beautiful," she said.

"Yeah."

"I'm sorry," Jamie said, her hand on my shoulder.

"Yeah."

"Here they come," she said, glancing out the unit window. Trina pushed Mom down the hallway as Dad and the family trotted behind them. Trina caught my eye over Mom's head, our greeting dire. Dad stared straight ahead.

We went back into the smelly on-call room. I shifted Lamonica to my left shoulder, our hearts touching. I could not infuse the strength of my heart into hers. I could not make her better. I could only hope to make these moments bearable. She was pinker and warm but breathing agonally—that is, dying slowly. The walls shut out the din of the unit. The only sounds I heard were Lamonica's wheezes and the blood rushing in my ears. I gave her to Grandma and left the room to give them privacy. I found Sharon again.

"Do I do something?"

"No. Let them be."

"This sucks." I folded my arms, petulant.

"Yes, it does. But they've got you."

"And I'm doing so much."

"You're doing more than you know."

I squinted at Sharon. I wasn't buying it.

When I returned, Lamonica lay in Grandma's arms. The family talked softly to each other. The air seemed calmer, almost peaceful.

"She's sleeping," Grandma whispered.

Silent, I checked for pulses and heart rate. None.

Dr. Manali, the doctor on call, waited outside the door. She came in and performed the same ritual.

"I'm so sorry," Dr. Manali said to the family. "She's gone."

Mom and Dad looked stone faced at their child. Their brief time as parents was over.

"She looks so peaceful," said Grandma.

"Yes, she does," I said.

"Twelve noon," Dr. Manali said to me, calling time of death. I blinked in acknowledgment.

Grandma passed Lamonica to Mom, who kissed her and passed her back to me. Dad kissed her. The family filed out of the room. I held her over my shoulder. She was still a warm bundle, just as she had been an hour ago. But she wasn't breathing. Her blood wasn't running through her. The pump had stopped. The chemical reactions and electrical impulses that were life itself had ended. She had lost, and we'd lost her.

Her family trudged down the hall. Dad pushed Mom, flanked by grandparents. They'd bent their heads. Sniffing and crying echoed off the concrete walls, the scuffed white linoleum, and the flickering fluorescent lights. They disappeared through the door, empty-handed, leaving their child in my arms.

I brought Lamonica back to her warming table. The nurses set up divider screens as a gesture of respect, giving us privacy from staff and other babies' parents and visitors. Postmortem care is not a show to see. It is a reminder of what can and does happen in an ICU.

Jamie had left paper and an inkpad on Lamonica's shelf. I took palm prints and footprints. As I filled a basin with warm water and a little baby soap, I kept looking at her monitor out of habit until I caught myself. I bathed her, smoothed lotion on her skin, and dressed her in a clean diaper.

I wrapped her up again. We left the unit and went to a small room tucked away near the on-call room. Inside and opposite a desk, a crib stood against the wall. I laid Lamonica inside and rummaged through the desk drawer for the camera. I fished it out and looked for the instructions.

This camera was special and for one specific use—postmortem pictures. We took the pictures, filled out a form, and sent the camera to the company. A few weeks later, the company sent us photos of the child. The pictures are hard to look at. The babies' eyes are closed. They are often puffy, and their skin is mottled blue, green, or gray; the pictures are obviously of dead babies. For many families, these will be their only baby pictures.

I'd watched another nurse use the camera once. I read the instructions. I looked at Lamonica. I looked at the camera. I looked at the clock. She had been my only assignment. Now that she was gone, I felt pushed to hurry up and get on to a new patient.

I spent the next fifteen minutes trying to make Lamonica look as comfortable and natural as possible. But the fluorescents were harsh. Her brown face had a blue tinge, and her closed eyes were puffy. I wondered if I was doing the right thing, but I took the pictures.

We returned to the unit. I snipped a lock of her hair and put it in a plastic bag. I picked out a pink bereavement box, in which I placed her footprints, her palm prints, the lock of hair, the measuring tape that showed her length, an extra armband with her name on it, her hat, and her name card. Somehow, this box would get to her parents. Mementos of their daughter's NICU stay. Tangible evidence of her life.

I had run out of things to do with her. It was time to call transport. A voice broke through my reverie.

"Diane? Have you eaten?"

It was Suzanne, a veteran nurse and our charge nurse for the day.

"No." It was two thirty.

"Why don't you go eat, and I'll finish with her," she said, motioning to Lamonica.

"I was just getting ready to call transport."

"I'll do it. You've had a long morning and you haven't had lunch. When you get back, you'll pick up Jamie's assignment when she leaves at three."

"You sure?"

"Yes. You've done what you can. I'll finish. Go."

I looked at pale brown Lamonica, cool on the table, secretly glad I didn't have to put her in a body bag. I silently thanked Suzanne.

"OK," I said and walked away.

· · ·

At seven thirty that evening, the setting sun dappled the canopy of trees along Sue's narrow street. Her townhouse was a historic building. A planter overflowing with herbs and ivy dominated the front stoop. Tall front windows beckoned. The house seemed dark at first, but the kitchen was bright and welcoming. Vanilla scented the air.

"Hi, honey," Sue said.

"Hey," I said, hoisting myself onto a kitchen stool. I took in the spread: cheeses, crackers, and olives. Van Morrison and Marvin Gaye crooned. Because I was single, my dinners often took place in front of the TV or over the sink. Eating at work was a joke—it was on the run or not at all. In my world, nourishment was a need not always honored.

Sue elevated the ordinary to extraordinary. I loved this ritual of entertaining. The set table, candles, and music—the commitment to being human, to sitting down and relaxing.

"The baby die?" Sue asked, chopping a red onion, not missing a lick.

I poured myself some wine and swirled the ruby liquid in the glass.

"Yeah. Around noon," I said, taking a sip. I told her the story. "After Mom goes upstairs, she codes, so Sharon and I are doing CPR. Jamie calls the floor, we get Mom back down . . ." I babbled.

"Oh, my God," said Sue.

"So they all hurry back," I continued. "This time I just left them and helped Jamie with a feed and some vital signs. When I came back, she was dead. Grandma thought she was sleeping."

"Well, she was . . ."

I rolled my eyes at her, taking another slug of wine. "I think I'm just realizing how awful those eight hours were."

"It's not easy."

"I wasn't sure what I was supposed to be doing."

"Sounds like you did it."

"Um. I didn't do much."

"More than you know. You going to Charlottesville tomorrow?" she said, changing the subject.

"Yeah."

"Heard from Dan?"

"No."

We moved outside. The warm September evening wrapped around me. After the unit's bright lights and noise, this was a cocoon whose dark quiet balanced the day. A gentle breeze brushed away its troubles. The patio sparkled in candles and starlight. Van, Marvin, and traffic mingled. My mind slowly settled. My breath evened out. I felt that hollow ache again, the ache I'd felt on the interstate before work. I wanted Dan here.

Over salad and steak, we kvetched about the unit, gossiped, and mulled my on-and-off romantic relationship, waxing philosophical on those matters best contemplated with wine and in darkness.

When I finally got home, angry feline eyes greeted me.

"Sorry, Phoebe," I said to my cat. Her black tail flicked as she led me into the kitchen. "You're going to be by yourself tomorrow too," I said, kissing the top of her head.

Two messages waited on my answering machine—one from my dad, the other from Karen, who'd left tomorrow's details along with a profuse apology for having called me at work. No call from Dan, but why would there be? I watched Phoebe eat. I thought of Leslie and Levon coming home with empty arms to an empty house. Dan seemed so trivial in comparison. I kissed Phoebe again.

Weeks went by. Dan returned. Turkeys and cornucopias decorated the unit's reception area. It was eight thirty in the evening. I'd gotten off at seven but hung around because I had patient notes to write and gabbing to do with Annie, our night receptionist, about her new boyfriend and my renewed one.

Two women, one older, one younger, entered the reception area. They approached the counter and peered over a flock of plastic turkeys. "We're looking for registration."

"Registration?" Annie and I said in unison. Their request was unusual; visitors said things like, "We're here to see Baby Clooney."

"Registration," they replied.

"For?" I asked. I sized them up. They were well dressed and well groomed. Neither looked pregnant. Annie and I looked at each other, as confused as the two women.

The younger woman said, "Someone called yesterday and said to come to registration to pick up pictures."

"Pictures?" I asked.

"Yes," she said.

"Pictures of?"

"Our baby girl. She died in September. Someone took pictures of her."

I sucked in my breath. "Lamonica."

"Yes, Lamonica. I'm Leslie, her mom."

I'd forgotten that I'd taken Lamonica's picture, that the pictures had come back yesterday. I'd forgotten that it had taken us fifteen minutes to remember who had died and when. I'd forgotten that another nurse was going to call the family about the pictures. I was disgusted with myself about all I had forgotten—a baby had died in my arms, and I'd pushed her out of my mind.

"Lamonica," I repeated. Images of the day rushed back—an ashen-faced woman with matted hair and a green hospital gown. A baby hat and onyx eyes in a cocoa-blue face. "I took those pictures. I was her nurse that day. Diane."

"Yes. I remember you."

"I'm so sorry I didn't recognize you. Yes, the pictures came yesterday. Suzanne called you." I fumbled through Annie's drawer, looking for the white cardboard envelope. "I wasn't sure if you wanted them, but I took them anyway, just in case."

I pulled the envelope from the drawer.

Mom and Grandma huddled together and opened it. They took out three pictures; Mom closed her eyes and smiled. Grandma put her arm around her daughter and kissed her head.

"Thank you so much," Leslie whispered.

"You're welcome," I said.

"Did you put the box together too?" she said.

"You got it? Yes, I did that."

"We did. Thank you. It was all such a blur. We're so grateful for the footprints and hair. And now, pictures."

I didn't know what to say.

Mom continued. "She was a surprise, you know," she said, stroking the picture.

"No, I didn't know."

"Yep. She wasn't planned. But she was a blessing, even for a day."

I stayed quiet.

Mom held out her arms and gestured a hug. "I'm so glad you're here tonight."

"Me too. I got off at seven, but I've been lollygagging for some reason," I said, hugging her. She smelled like cocoa butter and spice. "I'm glad you like the pictures. I feel like I didn't do much that day."

"You did a lot. You did," she said. She had one hand on my arm. She held her daughter's picture tight in the other hand.

"How's Dad?" I said.

"He's fine. We got married last month. We're good, everything is really good."

"You look wonderful. I'm so glad I was here to give you these."

"Me too. Thank you again for everything."

"No problem. Have a wonderful Thanksgiving."

"You too. Happy Thanksgiving."

Mom and Grandma waved one more time and smiled as they walked out the door.

Annie sniffed. We looked at each other in silence. I opened the unit door and watched them go, their heads together, still looking at the pictures. I felt Lamonica's swaddled body against my chest again, her soft hair on my cheek, her heart stirring against mine. I did not know, as I watched them leave, that I would more than make up for my inexperience in the next few weeks. Our NICU would face devastating losses: seven babies would die in a span of ten days. Five of them would be mine.

I would perform their postmortem care—bathe them, prepare them, make bereavement boxes, and take pictures. But they would have different experiences than Lamonica's. Those babies would die in the hands of strangers, albeit compassionate ones. Their deaths would be accompanied by frenzied codes, bright lights, cold air, crushing hands, and sharp needles trying to jab life into resistant bodies. Those babies would not die with ease among their families. They would not die in peace or quiet. I did not know, as I watched Leslie make her way down the hall, that she would be the only parent of a patient who died that I'd ever see again. I did not know what a gift she gave me.

Leslie and her mother reached the street door. They had almost disappeared. They walked the same hallway they had walked two months earlier. Same concrete walls. Same scuffed floor. Same overhead lights. But they stood straighter. Murmurs and laughter floated back to me. The white envelope caught the light as they left. Leslie's perfume clung to my scrubs top. That night, we did not leave the unit empty handed.

DIANE KRAYNAK *is a pediatric nephrology nurse practitioner. She is working on a collection of nursing essays, from which "Heart Lessons" is her third publication.*

DOCKING IN TOGO

Jennifer Binger, as told to Ann Swindell

A volunteer aboard a Mercy Ships vessel in Togo is overwhelmed by the country's extreme poverty and lack of medical resources yet unwavering in her commitment to individual patients.

I eyed the gol-ball-size growth on her foot. "*Douleur?*" I asked, using one of the few French words I knew. I needed to know if it caused pain.

"*Non,*" she shook her head. The grays in her black hair ran like railroad tracks from her temples.

I turned to the interpreter. "Ask her if it has grown at all in the last six months."

She shook her head again, and I looked again at the interpreter. "She says it has been the same for years."

It was my turn to shake my head. "*Je suis désolée.*"

Her face darkened. "Why you come?" Her English was slightly better than my French. She started clicking at me. "Why you come?" She threw her hands toward the sun, shaking down to her toes. "Why? You care only children!"

Right, I thought. *That's why I'm here, unpaid, in West Africa. Because I don't care.* I wasn't even going to try to explain our parameters to her. We did serve adults, hundreds of them, along with hundreds of children. "I'm very sorry, ma'am." I reached for her shoulder, trying to console her. She shrugged away from me, speaking in a language I didn't understand. The translator refused to look at me.

I watched as she walked away, trying to remember why I was here. The people waiting beyond the gated holding pen, where we did our initial screenings, filled my field of vision. Hundreds waited. Some, I knew, had walked for days to get to our hospital, docked in Lomé, Togo.

The hospital was an old Danish rail ferry, stripped to the bones and rebuilt as a functioning hospital with living quarters. Nearly four hundred people lived on board. The medical care we gave was completely free and offered through Mercy Ships, an NGO supported by donors across the globe. Every person who worked on the ship, whether a nurse, doctor, ship engineer, or custodian, was a volunteer.

I motioned to the next person in line. Nearly a month into my seven-month stint, I was no longer flinching at what I saw. I had seen it all. Clubbed feet by the hundreds, football-size hernias, countless contractures of fingers fused together by fire. Shoulders were fused to necks, wrists to forearms. Tumors dotted people like overgrown freckles. They bulged from eyes. They poured from mouths, bigger than softballs. We couldn't even consider a person for surgery if her tumor was smaller than an orange because so many people had tumors bigger than grapefruits.

We had more patients than we could ever serve.

A man came to me next, dropped his pants, and pointed to what looked like a hernia. He told the translator he'd had it for multiple months. Yes, I told him. Yes, we could help.

Next. I could see a mother carrying her son from ten yards away. He was probably eight, maybe nine years old, and too big for her to carry. She started talking to the translator immediately, pointing to the child's arms, head, and eyes. I knew already that the son had cerebral palsy. I could see all the signs, all the odd angles at which his body hung.

I shook my head no.

The translator told her that we could not help, but she shook her head back at me, pointing again to his head and eyes, tears pooling at the inside corners of hers. What she wanted, I couldn't explain to her, was the same thing any mother wants. She wanted a cure we didn't yet have. She wanted us to magically transform that broken little boy into someone whole.

She grabbed at my hand, held it on her son's head. "Please," she said. "Please."

I felt my throat contract. "There's nothing we can do. Even in America we can't fix this. I am so, so sorry."

The bodies continued to move toward and past me: a man with a tumor that restricted his ability to eat, too many babies with cleft palates to count. Keloids were common. Overgrowths of scar tissue that result from injuries and cuts, they piled like small mountains on the flesh and spread like a hot rash all over the body. They often grew on those with certain genetic tendencies and were usually exacerbated by the tribal scarring rituals that painted the bodies of both women and men. Then there was the hydrocephalus I saw nearly weekly—people with fluid on the brain, children with heads three times their normal size. They drooped under the weight of their own skulls.

Bowed legs, backward legs, knobby knees everywhere. The backward legs, bent like a chicken's, the knees inverted but not collapsing, were the hardest for my brain to comprehend.

Pain, disgrace, hurt, and confusion swirled around me on these days. I was thankful that I spent most of my time in wards with pediatric patients, watching most of them get better. But all nurses on the ship had to pay their screening dues. It was work that most of us could handle for only six or eight hours at a time.

I loved my work inside the ship but not out here. Out in the sun and behind the ridiculous gates, I had to say no more times than I could say yes. If a problem wasn't going to lead to death, infection, or dysfunction, I usually had to turn the person away. We could only help the really sick or terribly disfigured. There were so many of these souls that even our eight-month mooring in the country could not serve them all.

Inside the ship, though, I always got to say yes. *Yes, you can have more food. Yes, you can drink more water. Yes, your body is healing. Yes, you will be able to go back home without being an outcast. Yes, the tumor is going away. Yes, you will be able to walk normally. Yes, your child will live.* Inside the ship, my whole life was a yes. *Yes, we can fix your brokenness. Yes, I can help you see normally. Yes, yes, yes. Yes, my life matters here.*

Yes, my life mattered on the ship. That was why I'd come, why I had long wanted to come to this ship and give medical care to the poorest of the poor. When I started to imagine becoming a nurse during my time in college, seven years ago, this was always in the back of my mind. If I were going to be a nurse, I was going to work for Mercy Ships. It seemed romantic and raw, and I could learn a skill and help to save lives; it was that simple. At a place like Mercy Ships, the wards were filled with people who had nowhere else to turn. I wanted to work at the end of the line. I wanted my life to matter.

After nursing school, I lacked the requisite two years of experience for Mercy Ships, so I volunteered in Jinja, Uganda, for three months before returning to the States to start my first paid job, on a pediatric floor in northern Illinois. As soon as I finished two years of active nursing, I turned in my application. Mercy Ships accepted me, and I quit my job, packed a duffel, and took a flight to the Canary Islands, where the *Africa Mercy* had been getting a much-needed tune-up. We then sailed down to the thin strip of land sandwiched between Benin and Ghana—the country of Togo. Lomé, the capital city, was our docking port.

Togo is heartbreakingly poor, fitting almost every stereotype that Americans have of Africa. It is a nation of more than six and a half million people, with over half of the population at or below the poverty line. Children do starve here, and people die of AIDS every day. Doctors are rare. Good medical care is rarer. This is why Mercy Ships docks in Togo regularly. It's accessible, the government is willing, and the people need care desperately.

Almost a quarter of the staff of *Africa Mercy* volunteered year-round. By fundraising for themselves, they were able to work on the ship as full-time doctors, technicians, nurses, or even teachers for the children who lived aboard. The rest of us came as seasonal volunteers, paying our own ways. Crew fees were due every month and helped to cover the costs of lodging, food, and the operation of the ship. Many volunteers were Christian, as Mercy Ships was and continues to be a faith-based organization. But the only indispensable qualification was a desire to help.

Tani was incredibly small for an eight-year-old, so small that our children's gowns slipped off her shoulders. Boiling water had burned off her nose and disintegrated her right ear and right eye. Her right hand was only partially functional. She had been two or three years old when she was burned, we guessed, because she remembered nothing of her life with two eyes.

It looked as if a grenade had exploded on her tiny face. Her black skin had turned pinkish-white at the temple, and the pigment above her eye had been permanently burned away. Her ear was a tiny hole surrounded only by a spiral of skin that warped around it like a snake. Whatever pot of water had fallen on her must have been scathingly hot. She had survived an accident that would have killed most toddlers.

She spoke a language so obscure that we would have to use at least three translators at a time to understand her. French was the official language in Togo, although many people spoke tribal languages as well or better. But patients who came from the bush spoke any number of languages, and Tani spoke something that none of our hired translators understood. Her life, to us, was a mystery.

Life in medicine comes with its own language, and life on a medical ship creates its own type of reality. Our speech was infused with nautical terms and hospital lingo. Physical space was understood in terms of decks, wards, and berths. The hospital was on deck three; living quarters were on decks three and four. Deck seven had an outdoor play area for younger patients and the best view of the water and the city. I lived on deck three; our living cabins were beyond a fire door just past the hospital. My cabin was a six berth, meaning that six people lived in it. My cabin door opened to a thin hallway that unfolded into three cubicles, each of which contained a bunk bed that two people shared. Behind the flimsy curtain in the second cubicle in cabin 3418—bottom bunk—was where I lived for the seven months I was on the ship.

The entire time we were in Togo, the nurses, doctors, and other volunteers came and went; some came for as little as two weeks, while others started two-year stints.

I came to know the nurses best, of course. We were a mix of men and women from all over the world. English was the common language on the ship, so most of us were American, Canadian, Australian, or New Zealander, with a handful of Europeans tossed in.

When my first roommate left in April, Beth became my new bunkmate. From California, she was slim, blond, and brilliant; she was also ragingly sick the entire time she was on the *Africa Mercy*. As we all learned, sickness was an unfortunate but common side effect of life for first-world immune systems in Africa. The immunizations, shots, and medications we took could not protect our fragile bodies from everything. The doctors on the ship discovered a parasite in Beth's body, and when she was finally starting to recover, a coconut fell from a palm tree overhead, smashing her ankle as she rested by the waterline. I found her back in our bunk with an ice pack on her foot.

"At least it didn't hit my head," she laughed.

"At least the medical care is free," I offered in return. "I'm so sorry, Beth."

Her eyes sharpened. "Let's be honest, Jen. What I'm dealing with is nothing like what people in Togo live with. I'll be fine."

Tani's voice was a whistle, high and piercing. I never understood anything she said, but the other pediatric unit nurses and I tried to teach her the little French we knew. Her voice was unmistakable, even in its untranslatable consonants. It hung in the air, then dipped like a flung yo-yo when she laughed. And she laughed constantly: she laughed when we had to change her dressings, marveling at the gauze and its lightness; she laughed and held my hand while singing to me; and as often as she could, she would laugh while stealing me away to deck seven, where we would play Go Fish or ride tricycles together. Her crooked smile was always just below the surface of her plasticky skin, waiting to erupt.

This was the unshakeable thing about Tani: she was happy. Actually happy. I wasn't sure that she realized how abnormal she looked, how different she was. Her easy joy challenged me, helping to keep me from the self-pity that lived at the edge of an uncomfortable situation. Yes, I lived in a tiny bunk bed on a ship in Africa with no personal space. *But if she can smile*, I kept telling myself, *then I can suck it up. I can do this. This is not hard. This is joy, helping people live.*

This, I started to believe, was why I was alive. To help others live.

O'Brian joined our pediatric unit while Tani was in the middle of her surgery and recovery cycle. A three-month-old boy who came to us weighing only five pounds, his ribs played on his skin like old guitar strings, completely visible and ready to break. His mother brought him to the ship because he had a bilateral cleft palate.

Our ship did dozens of cleft lip and palate surgeries every month, but a child must weigh at least ten pounds to have the operation. So we put O'Brian on our infant feeding program and weighed him every day. He couldn't latch well to his mother's breast, partly because of his cleft palate. We taught her to express milk in order to feed him. When O'Brian wouldn't take the expressed milk, we gently ran a feeding tube down his tiny throat.

His mother was quiet, staying constantly by his side. On his good days, he would gain an ounce or two.

"He's doing well today. He is gaining strength."

She could hear, in the pitch of my voice, the sound of hope that depends not on one's language but on one's desire.

She nodded, smiling back. The tribal scars under her eyes ran in straight lines down to her mouth; when she smiled, they tightened. She would often put her hand on O'Brian's head and just hold it there.

Sometimes I tried talking to her in my broken French. *"D'autres enfants?"*

She looked down. *"Non."* O'Brian was her only child.

The doctors tried to re-create a nose for Tani. The hole in the middle of her face was not her most important medical need, but it was incredibly significant culturally. In Africa, people with any sort of physical mutation are often considered outcasts, cursed; they are unwanted. A nose was important for her survival because it could mean better care from her parents and others. It meant that she might be able to go to school. So the nose was first. The doctors were able to graft skin from her head to form a "nose" that— despite looking a bit like the end of a rolled cigar—gave a human silhouette to her face. She giggled over the little patches of fuzz that grew on her nose for the first few weeks—hair from her head that replaced itself on the bridge of her new nose that would never work.

That surgery was followed by another, in which the doctors took a skin flap from the side of her head and grafted it to her face to create a more regular mouth shape. Skin from her thigh was then grafted to her cheek to help create an eye socket. Although she would never again see out of that eye, the goal was to create a secure space where a prosthetic could eventually be positioned.

Skin and muscle grafts require incredibly sterile dressings, and each one takes at least two weeks to heal. So after the nose surgery, she had weeks of healing time. Once that skin was healthy enough, the doctors labored on her mouth and her eye socket. She was constantly sore, dripping from some wound, wearing some sort of bandage.

Her bad eye was weepy; although it had been completely burned, she still had a tear duct. Whenever she sneezed, the duct would seep without fail. Her little sneezes would ricochet off the metal beds and handrails in the pediatric ward. "Tani!" Beth would laugh. "Use your tissues." We had given Tani a little packet of them to carry, and Beth would pretend to wipe her own eye, then point to Tani. "Wipe your eye."

She would bob her head at us, wipe the gooey liquid away, then skip over to the trash cans to deposit her tissues.

"Way to go, Tani," I would tell her. She would run to her bed, giggling. *Only one eye*, I thought . *But that good eye sparkles.*

The bathroom in our cabin was four feet square, including the sink, toilet, and shower. We were allowed a total of two minutes of water each day on the ship, so I learned the art of showering dry. Wet my hair, turn the water off, shampoo, turn the water on. Repeat with soap. Pray the air conditioning didn't flip on while you were showering. Pray it turned on while you were working your shift, when the sweat was sliding down your back and through your scrubs.

After two months, O'Brian started to develop breathing problems. He was stalling out at six pounds and, we discovered, aspirating some of the milk we desperately wanted him to eat. Oxygen therapy didn't help, so we tried to fashion a tiny continuous positive airway pressure (CPAP) mask for his little face in order to keep his airways open.

His mother could tell that he was not getting better. She was worried, anxious. Once in a while, another nurse and I would offer to pray for her and O'Brian. As we bowed our heads together, I never knew if she understood our meaning but on more than one occasion, we looked up from the short prayers to find each other's faces wet with tears.

I once stopped by O'Brian's bed during a night shift to watch him breathe. His mother slept next to him, always close. Despite all our care, he would not—or could not—put on the weight necessary for his surgery. He was nearly six months old and still significantly shy of ten pounds. I knew he would not make it.

Tani loved to have her nails painted; I had brought several bottles of nail polish in my duffel, and I'd learned that pediatric patients loved to watch the colors on my fingers fly as I reapplied their dressings or fixed their IV drips.

I was painting Tani's nails during one of my breaks one afternoon. I looked at her straight on, this little girl with half a face, a fuzzy nose, and an unstoppable smile. I found myself thanking God for not letting that boiling water kill her.

"I love you, Tani." I meant it. "You're beautiful." I meant that too.

She spoke back to me, always a mystery.

I repeated what I'd said. "I love you. You're beautiful."

She looked at me, and I said it a third time.

She started to parrot me, the high C of her voice bouncing: "I love you, Tani. You're beautiful." Her accent was thick, but the English words worked in her mouth.

"If you want to say it about yourself, say, '*I'm* beautiful.'"

She repeated, "I love you Tani I'm beautiful I love you Tani I'm beautiful." She was now giggling, smearing the pink nail polish on her little blue gown. "I love you I'm beautiful! I love you I'm beautiful!"

I started laughing, too. She had no idea what she was saying.

She pointed to me, the signal that she wanted me to talk.

"Yes, Tani. I love you. You're beautiful."

One of my favorite times of the week came on Sunday, when we held Ward Church. It was a respite from the normal rhythm of weekly ward life, something different in the midst of all the surgeries and dressings and bed pans. Patients were not required to go, but most of them did. I imagined that they were tired of staring at the same walls every day.

They came down the hallways clutching their drool rags, NG tubes hanging out of their noses, little pouches from their drains pinned to their gowns and flapping on their hips. Multiple patients scooted down the hallways in wheelchairs, or they walked while wheeling IV tubes beside them. Every single patient came to church in a blue gown, their standard attire. I loved that most of the women wore colorful wraps around their waists. In a sea of blue, their reds, purples, and greens showed up beautifully.

We would try to fit seventy five of us—patients, nurses, doctors, custodians, cooks, ship engineers—in C ward, which held twenty bunk beds. Patients sat on each other's beds, held each other's children, held each other's IVs. The service started with music, usually with bongo drums and the translators singing in French. African worship on the ship was always full of wholehearted dancing; it was nothing like the stoic hymns I'd sung in church as a kid. And it went on and on, the sick and seeping who danced, swayed, and sweated, following each other in circles, full of laughter and shouts. The dancers' gowns flapped in the thick air, and the clapping was loud despite the drool rags held by many, which muted the sound. I joined in whenever I could, sweating through my scrubs, my blond hair sticking to my neck.

We danced, sang, sweated, and laughed for as long as the patients had energy; sometimes half an hour, sometimes forty-five minutes. After a sermon from a translator or one of the ship's volunteers, we would dance and sing again. We all loved this opportunity to dance freely and together, to mold a second relationship besides patient and doctor, sick and caretaker. We were on the same plane here, the languages melting together into laughter and praise that needed no particular tongue to be understandable. We all knew that we needed more help than our own hands could offer. Seeing the babies with the cleft palates healing, the faces with the tumors receding, the grafted skin re-growing, the cataracts clearing, I saw church for the first time in my life.

I was taking a day off to explore Lomé on the day O'Brian died. The ship sent a car for me because his mother wanted me to see him and to say good-bye.

I got back to the ship and met with her in a side room. She was holding O'Brian. He was out of his hospital gown, dressed by the nursing staff in baby clothes that actually fit. The yellow onesie was bright against his skin and soft around the sleeves. O'Brian looked peaceful, the little hint of a baby smile at the left corner of his mouth. I went to hug her, and she held me, each of us crying, sharing the only language in which we had ever communicated fluently.

I knew that her return to her village with a dead son held grievous consequences not only for her heart but also for her social status. She had to go back home to her husband without a son. All of our work at the hospital had been useless; by the time she had been able to get to us, he had deteriorated so much that there was practically nothing we could do. If we could have gotten to him sooner, maybe things would have been different.

She shook her head, embraced me again, and had to leave. She would carry her dead son back to her village to bury him.

Since our patient numbers were down during our last week in Togo, we let Tani play on the ward floors. More than anything, she loved punching the numbers on the ship phones and making "calls" to other parts of the ship. She mimicked the doctors and nurses who made calls all day; most of her dials ended up going nowhere, but she rattled into the phone like the rest of us did.

One afternoon, I came back to my cabin and actually had a message from Tani. She had repeated, "I love you I'm beautiful I love you I'm beautiful!" into the answering machine. I wanted to rip the phone off the wall and carry it away it in my backpack.

And when I landed in Chicago, my first thought was how I would get back to the ship before it sailed again, three months later.

O'Brian and Tani had marked me deeply. One died, one lived. Pediatric nursing is not easy. The outcome isn't always what you've hoped for a child. But I still nurse, near Chicago, for children dying of cancer and those living through it, for kids struggling through pneumonia and those having asthma attacks. Life. Death. Nursing has forced me to realize that I don't determine if someone makes it or not. I can try to help. But I cannot always give the one thing I've been trained to give, the one thing I want to give: healing.

I was covering an ER shift for a friend, several weeks ago, when a woman was brought in by Social Services.

"The old lady pooped everywhere, Jen. I need your help in room three." I grimaced as Katie passed me. "I'll be there in a second," she said. "Need to grab a few supplies."

I closed my eyes and took a deep breath, then pushed the door open.

"Hello," I said. "How are you?"

She gestured with her hands and spoke in a voice as stringy as seaweed. I had no clue what she was telling me. She was anxious, cautious. She was probably seventy.

"I'm sorry, but I don't know what you're saying." I tried to communicate with my facial expressions. "We're going to get you cleaned up." Whatever language she was speaking was something I'd never heard before.

Katie walked in with some washcloths. I turned to her. "What language does she speak?"

"No clue," she shrugged. "The only interpreter we have available tonight is for Spanish."

I shook my head. "That's definitely not it."

My guess was an Eastern European dialect. But it was two in the morning, and I wasn't sure how coherent she was. The patient leaned back in her bed, the remains of her orange hair sticking to the pillow that was propped under her back and shoulders. She started mumbling.

I looked at the chart. Aside from her name, we hardly knew anything. There was a huge lump on her arm; based on the X-ray, it looked like she had suffered a broken bone weeks ago. Katie and I gloved up and started to clean her, careful to avoid putting any pressure on her arm. This is half of my job, cleaning up the messes bodies make.

She watched me the whole time, looking at me longer than she should have. She had apparently given up on trying to communicate verbally. I finally looked back at her, as I was putting the sheet over her chest, and saw the age spots on her heavy skin, the confusion in her huge, dark eyes.

She suddenly grabbed my hand and pulled it toward her mouth. I was afraid she was going to bite me, so I gently pulled it away and continued cleaning her body. But she again tried to pull my hand, and when I let her, she kissed it. I softened and looked at her.

"You're welcome," I said.

She kissed my hand again.

"You're welcome," I said one more time, looking at her eyes. And then I was looking at O'Brian, looking at Tani.

I love you, I thought. *You're beautiful.*

JENNIFER BINGER *lives in Wheaton, Illinois, and is a full-time pediatric nurse. She is also a part-time women's college soccer coach.*

ANN SWINDELL *received her MFA from Seattle Pacific University and teaches writing courses at Wheaton College. She lives west of Chicago with her husband and has written for multiple anthologies, magazines and websites, including Halogentv.com and Relevantmagazine.com.*

I SEE YOU

Tilda Shalof

After being conscripted to care for her family throughout her childhood, a young woman goes into nursing as a means of escape. She is pleasantly surprised to discover the camaraderie and rewarding work of the ICU—and to find a second career as a writer.

> Cherry, being a nurse, felt sympathy for all living creatures.
> —Helen Wells, *Cherry Ames, Camp Nurse*

Good for you, Nurse Cherry Ames, but that's not me. Not in the early days, at least.

Guinness World Records, please take note: I hold the record for youngest nurse ever: I was born a nurse. Even as an infant, I sensed it was expected of me to care for others. Never mind that I didn't want to do so, nor was I particularly good at it. As a toddler, I stayed close to my depressed, invalid mother, helping her with her every move and trying to cheer her up. As a child, I monitored my father's diabetes, administered his insulin, and ran for his nitroglycerin tablets whenever he had chest pains. All the while, I did my best to soothe the psychotic storms and paranoid rages of my schizophrenic brother. I took care of them all, dutifully in my youth but resentfully in my angry and rebellious teenage years. By the time I decided to apply to nursing school, I was wild, undisciplined, and self-absorbed. In short, everything you wouldn't want in a nurse.

Unlike Cherry Ames, iconic nurse of the novels bearing her name, I had no "desire to help people." Published mostly in the 1940s and '50s, the series was already becoming outdated by the time I read the books in the '70s. She was selfless, angelic, and compassionate. I was, well . . . not. For me, "desire to help people" was just a phrase for sincere and earnest candidates to put down on their nursing school applications. I was unsuited to care for a hamster, much less sick people. Nor did I wish to do so, thank you very much, after having spent my entire childhood in the starring role of de facto nurse for the variously ill, depressed, deranged, and malingering members of my own family.

When I chose nursing, I was running toward the exact thing I'd wanted to escape. Nursing was comfortable and familiar, on the one hand—a no-brainer. But I was fed up with sickness, infirmity, and disease. I longed for adventure, freedom, romance—*What better way to meet those goals than a career in nursing?* I reasoned. Perhaps, like Cherry, I could be a Dude Ranch Nurse, a Ski Patrol Nurse, or a Tropical Cruise Nurse and have glamorous and exciting adventures. Best of all, nursing would be my ticket to independence; it would provide me a livelihood and an escape from the dreariness of home. Yes, I did want to be kind and compassionate like Cherry and the nurses whom I'd observed caring for my parents during their various hospitalizations. But caring for others didn't come naturally to me. I had to work at it. Grudgingly, I hoped that nursing would remediate me, correct me, tame my wild side. No, I didn't like caring for sick people, but it felt noble to do so. Besides, people always told me, "You look like a nurse." They meant sweet, gentle, and kind, which I am, mostly. *Don't become a nurse, don't become a nurse,* I told myself. What did I do? I became a nurse. My heart wasn't in it. My heart was hardened against it.

I took the first job that came my way after graduation, on a general medicine floor. I was completely unprepared. As a new, university-educated nurse, I had been instructed to "assist our patients on their journeys of self-actualization." I was there to "maximize wellness" through the "therapeutic use of myself." I was going to be a "change agent," a "nursing leader," and a "holistic healer." I felt an ongoing tension between the university-educated nurses like me and the old guard, the hospital-trained nurses. Maybe those veterans didn't know much about research or nursing theories, but they sure knew how to care for patients. They got the job done. I wanted to be like them—a nurse who could start IVs on anyone; a nurse who confidently flicked air bubbles out of IV tubing; one who placed defibrillator paddles on the patient's chest and called out, "Stand back!"

I had six patients on my first day. Someone had a low urine output and needed a Foley catheter; I had read about this procedure but had never performed it. I looked at the long list of meds to give, vital signs to take, dressings to change, IVs to monitor, and fluid balances to tally. And, of course, there was a mountain of charting to do. Change agent? Nursing leader? I was just trying to survive and make it through my shift without killing anyone. All the theories, conceptual frameworks, and research methodologies I'd learned at the university were useless to me; I needed physical stamina and a thick skin. Resilience, self-control, and common sense would have helped too. I had none of these qualities. It seemed as if my sole activity was to respond to the endlessly ringing call bells. I felt like one of Pavlov's dogs. Before I could run to meet one patient's needs, another bell would already be calling me from another direction and toward someone else's distress.

Caring for patients was difficult enough, but dealing with the nurses was worse. They were hard on me, out to get me—or so I thought. I was a tuna in a shark tank, swimming ferociously, trying to evade the predators. At the beginning of every shift, I wondered when and how they would attack. I have since learned that there is such a thing as a nurse shark in marine life, and I swear I met its human counterparts on that general medicine floor. As for the patients? They were plankton. Mere algae. I was supposed to offer them comfort and safety, but I had none to spare.

I was treading water, desperate to stay afloat. The other nurses huddled together, whispering, gossiping, tut-tutting, and rolling their eyes. They criticized me for doing my work too slowly or too quickly, for being too disorganized, messy, and inefficient. I didn't argue with them because they were right.

"You bulldozed ahead to change the patient's bed, but he's been discharged."

"You dumped the urine! Did you forget about the twenty-four-hour collection?"

One day, I entered a patient's room and found him prone and still. I ran for the crash cart, panicked, calling for a code blue. By the time everyone had rushed into my room, my patient had sat up and yawned. He'd been sleeping and wondered what all the commotion was about. Good for him, but embarrassing for me.

"Sure, she has book smarts," they allowed, "but she'll never make it here with that fancy university degree of hers. What are they teaching those university grads? They don't know a thing about patient care . . ."

They were right. I never made it there, and an escape route eventually presented itself.

One day, after having stuck it out on that brutal floor for almost a year, I sat in a nursing supervisor's office, moaning and sobbing. The work was too much for me, I said. I couldn't cope, I blubbered. "It's so upsetting," I cried, "seeing such sick people." Such an evident observation, but I had no idea how to handle my emotions.

"You're very sensitive, my dear," she said. "You have to learn how to get in and how to get out." I had no idea what she was talking about. But to avoid losing me (or perhaps simply to shut me up), she made an offer. "How would you like to work in the ICU?" I'd noticed the sign that pointed toward the ICU beside the elevators I took to get to my floor every day. For some reason, the letters registered in my brain as "I See You" as she spoke them. That statement beckoned me. It pointed me in a specific direction and seemed to possess a magical power, as if I were being seen and chosen. I had no idea whether working in the ICU would be any better than working on the floor, but it surely couldn't be any worse. "Good-bye," I said on the day I left. *Good riddance*, they must have thought. I thought the same about them.

On my first day in the ICU, a nurse cheerfully approached me. "Welcome to the House of Horrors," she said. At least she greeted me.

Compared to the soul-destroying smackdown of general medicine, the ICU was a heartwarming embrace. The work was fascinating and, most of all, fun. Initially, it was intimidating; these patients were *sick*. They had life-threatening illnesses, catastrophic conditions that affected every organ of their bodies. All were on life support, and their conditions could change in minutes. You had to be constantly alert, ready to take swift action. Espionage helped. I spied on the others, and what I admired, I copied. When I saw a nurse take a short cut or act sloppily or lazily, I vowed never to do the same. I ended up working with a group of nurses who became close friends as well as colleagues. We worked hard and partied hearty, too, staying out late and crawling into work the next morning. Or we'd work all night, go for breakfast in the morning, and talk about all the funny or sad, troubling or satisfying things that had happened on the night shift. By talking through it, we could put it all to bed and then, heading off to sleep the day away, do the same with our weary selves.

The skills of critical care nursing were challenging to learn but more easily achieved than the requisite emotional maturity. I was of no use to a young woman whose husband was diagnosed with leukemia six weeks into their marriage. "I'm so afraid of waking up next to a corpse," she said, sobbing. I could only gasp at her pain. Newly married myself, I identified with her so completely that I could only think, *I hope this never happens to me*; after I finished caring for her dying husband that day, I rushed home to make passionate love to my healthy one. In those days, there was no separation between me and my patients.

The ICU made me a nurse less by its machines and technological advancements than by its people and their expertise. The ICU is a way of doing things, a striving for excellence, an attention to detail. In the ICU, I discovered the possibility to become a masterful nurse. I remember a fresh postop patient who was shivering. *Was he going into hypovolemic shock? Was it anxiety? A possible seizure? Early signs of sepsis? A blood transfusion reaction?* I stood frozen as the possibilities crowded my mind. An experienced ICU nurse took over, assessed him, figured out the problem, and solved it. I yearned to be that nurse.

For the past twenty-five years, I have worked in the Medical-Surgical Intensive Care Unit at Toronto General Hospital. I have taken care of people as they took their first breaths with a new set of transplanted lungs or as a beloved family member died. Recently, my patient was a twenty-one-year-old man with cystic fibrosis who had received a lung transplant two days earlier. He was unstable, needing high concentrations of oxygen. His heart rhythm was irregular, and his urine output was minimal. His blood pressure was low. I knew that if I did anything incorrectly, if I didn't do something I should've done, or if I did something I shouldn't have done, he could die. I found it exhilarating. I knew I could help to make this man better, maybe even save his life. I worked hard and nonstop, and at the end of my shift, he'd made progress, much of which was the direct result of my care.

I'm often asked, "Isn't nursing depressing?" I have experienced real depression in my life, but not because of my profession. Nursing is the opposite of despair; it offers the opportunity to do something about suffering. But you have to be strong to be a nurse. You need strong muscles and stamina for the long shifts and heavy lifting, intelligence and discipline to acquire knowledge and exercise critical thinking. As for emotional fortitude—well, I'm still working on that. Most of all, you need moral courage because nursing is about the pursuit of justice. It requires you stand up to bullies, to do things that are right but difficult, and to speak your mind even when you are afraid. I wasn't strong like this when I started out. Nursing made me strong.

A few years ago, my career took a surprising turn. I was a nurse, wife, and hockey mom to two young sons, and in my spare time I loved to write. One night in the ICU, a doctor happened to mention, "Hospital stuff is hot. People want to know what really goes on in the hospital."

Who better than a nurse to tell them? I thought. I printed my stories and stuffed them into a plastic grocery bag. In the morning, I changed out of my scrubs and into jeans and a sweatshirt, walked to the office of McClelland and Stewart, Canada's top publishing house, and dropped them into the box marked In at the front desk. Within two days, they called to offer me a book contract.

"It's something new," the editor said, "a perspective you never hear."

He meant a nurse's voice. We are quiet, sometimes silent altogether. Every nurse knows these stories, but they'd never before found their way into print. I had witnessed so many things that I felt I couldn't say to anyone but another nurse. I rarely tell non-nurses or family members much about what I do. I keep it from them.

Nursing can be an extreme sport, and my stories are hardcore, with few miracles and no heroes or angels. I, for one, am neither heroic nor angelic; the nurses I know—hardworking, intelligent professionals doing incredibly challenging work—are no angels either.

It's easy to sentimentalize or underestimate the importance of nursing. This became clear to me when I once heard a patient speak about the nurse who had cared for her during her heart attack: "She was so sweet. She held my hand and never left my side. What an angel." In addition to holding the patient's hand, that nurse had analyzed her twelve-lead electrocardiogram and monitored her for arrhythmias. She had drawn serum troponin levels and ensured that electrolyte levels were normalized. She had given information, oxygenation, anticoagulation, and pain relief. When nurses speak about their work, we mostly mention the emotional aspects of it but not the skills we possess, our scientific knowledge, or patient outcomes. That's why I avoid popular slogans like Nurses make a difference. We do much more than that. Nurses heal people. We improve and even fix things. Nurses make *all* the difference—between safety and danger, life and death, and getting better or not.

It felt scary to tell my story. As I worked on my book, I knew by my physiological reactions that I was taking a risk: I would often get tachypneic, tachycardiac, diaphoretic; it would take courage to see this through. What was so dangerous? I wrote about the instances when I was more caught up with my own problems than those of my patients; the situations when I tried to be nonjudgmental and empathetic but wasn't; the day a patient told me he didn't want me to be his nurse. I confessed the errors I'd made. I wrote a lot about death, how we go too far to prolong our patients' lives, and how dreadful it feels to carry out treatments that offer no benefit, that even inflict pain and indignity. I wrote about the exhausting night shifts and the cups of black coffee and the bowls of popcorn at the nursing station that got us through them. I even wrote about a taboo: nurses' real feelings about dealing with poo and pee. Incontinence is hard for patients as well as for the nurses who at times feel defined by it. I wanted to tell how I ceased to feel demeaned by that aspect of my role and began to feel proud of my ability to help patients feel clean and dignified.

Nursing scholars tend to focus on evidence-based practice, but practice-based evidence has its place too. My stories are true accounts of the gutsy, smart, take-charge nurses I know: a nurse who analyzes arterial blood gases, diagnoses a metabolic acidosis, and knows how to correct it; a nurse who anticipates a cardiac arrest and prepares emergency drugs in syringes, just in case; a nurse who gently guides a family into the ICU on a first visit to a critically ill loved one—and who catches them when they fall back in shock and disbelief; a nurse who questions a doctor's order when it is inappropriate for the patient.

A Nurse's Story went into foreign translation, and now I hear from readers all over the world who want to know what nursing is all about. Every opinion poll says people have trust in and respect for nurses, yet they don't know what we do or the responsibilities we shoulder.

What is nursing? It is a force for goodness, a way to repair the world, a path toward the creation of caring communities. Nursing is my profession and my way of life. By having first found compassion for my own suffering, I can offer compassion to others. Nursing has given me awareness of the world's suffering, and it has shown me how to love things I thought I never could. It has expanded my vision exponentially: when I look at the world, all roads seem to lead to nursing. Every problem we face in our society— war, famine, poverty, crime, natural disasters, global warming—affects health and safety. The real-life human consequences of these challenges have nursing solutions. Where there's no peace, there's no health; if there is no safety, there is no health. Nurses know this and possess the knowledge and skills to ameliorate all of these situations. There is no issue that does not involve nursing. Any discussion about healthcare that doesn't involve nursing is inherently flawed. And nurses need to speak up more often and more loudly. Our voices will be heard only if we express them.

It took me a long time to see this bigger picture of nursing. For years, I saw nursing through a microscope—patient to patient, shift to shift. I can now take it all in with a telescope and see the long view of nursing as a way to repair the world.

I was timid and silent when I was a young nurse. I used to enter patients' room sideways, hoping to pass unnoticed, to do no harm. Now I know I have much to offer my patients and my profession. I was nothing like this when I started out, but nursing gave me my identity and my voice. Now I can't keep quiet.

"You've been taking care of patients for almost thirty years," my friends often note. (My closest friends know it's been longer than that!) "Isn't it time to move on to something bigger and better?"

"What could be better than this?" I answer.

Yes, I'm still in the ICU, caring for individuals and their families, still wanting to hear their stories and see deeply into their lives. I was the world's youngest nurse, once. I'm now aiming to be its oldest.

TILDA SHALOF *has been a nurse for nearly thirty years. She is the author of the best-selling* A Nurse's Story, *which has been translated into four languages;* The Making of a Nurse; Camp Nurse; *and* Opening My Heart—A Journey from Nurse to Patient and Back Again. *She still works in the Medical-Surgical Intensive Care Unit at Toronto General Hospital.*

LISTENING
and Other Lifesaving Measures

Karla Theilen

A recent graduate travels to a small hospital on a Navajo reservation in Arizona to begin her first job. Vexed by the hospital's systemic problems and facing burnout, she seeks advice from a friend and former mentor.

I stopped at a gas station to freshen up when I reached Tuba City. The wind whipped up the front of my skirt as I opened the car door, and I stepped hurriedly into the parking lot, piercing the uneaten portion of a hamburger bun with my sensible heel. I began to suspect I'd overdressed for the interview. In the restroom, I splashed water on my face, turning the red dust into little pink trickles that I wiped away with the back of my hand as they ran down my cheeks. It was no use. Driving across the red expanse of high desert had felt like an attempt to navigate a windstorm on Mars—in a golf cart. But despite the western gale, I'd felt myself being pulled toward the Navajo reservation in northeastern Arizona, driven by a much greater force than the Barbie-size rental car I'd picked up at the Phoenix airport, and I decided to give in.

A short distance from the gas station, I saw a hospital with three flags flying high: the American flag, the Arizona flag, and what I would come to recognize as the official flag of the Navajo Nation. This is where I had arranged to meet the nurse recruiter. "Turn into the east parking lot at the sign that says Emergency," he'd said, "and you'll see me there, by the flagpole."

I nearly drove past the wooden sign with Emergency stenciled across it in red capital letters. The tiny rental car bottomed out in a rut at the entrance to the parking lot, scattering a couple of scrawny stray dogs that had been fighting over what appeared to be a discarded slice of pizza. I thought about

Chancellor Drake's speech at the dismal graduation luncheon, months earlier, in which he'd apologetically deemed 2009 to be "the worst job market for new nurses since 1983." Nevertheless he had faith in us, he gushed, faith that if anyone could do it, it was our little class of nineteen students who had what it took to plow through an accelerated, fifteen-month bachelor of science in nursing (BSN) program. He was optimistic that his shining stars could travel to the ends of the earth, if need be, for their first nursing jobs. He was right, I thought, as I paused to take a deep breath before stepping out into the wind. For if Tuba City was not the end of the earth, it was within shouting distance.

The lone figure beside the flagpole waved as I teetered across the rutted dirt parking lot. He exuberantly shook my hand and put a lanyard with a name badge around my neck, my name spelled almost correctly and followed by the letters *RN*, which suggested that a successful interview was accomplished by simply showing up. "Sometimes people get to the parking lot and they just turn around. But we're working on it," he said with conviction, "on all of this." He extended his arm and made a grand, sweeping gesture. A candy wrapper, suspended magically on the wind, hovered for a moment before it dropped right in front of his feet. He stepped on it as we walked toward the hospital doors.

The hospital itself was an unimpressive one-story building with an old smell and a heavy feeling. The tour was brief. We moved quickly while he expounded on the proposed improvements and upgrades, as well as the state-of-the-art equipment that would be arriving any day—or at least within the year. He focused on recent accomplishments: the digital shift clock, the new IV pumps, an employee fitness center. He introduced me to nurses who seemed friendly, none of whom mouthed the words *don't do it* behind the nurse recruiter's back. Nor did they warn me with their hands by making the universal sign for choking or the one for shooting oneself in the head.

As we sat in his office negotiating the contract, he cleared his throat to assure me, in case I'd heard otherwise, that a few small problems had recently been fixed. For one, changing the security code on the side entrance, he said, had stopped the drunks from coming in during the middle of the night. And the tribal police had begun to crack down on the vandalism and burglaries at the residences of hospital employees. Although I would have to stay in a condo with several other nurses for a while, he assured me that it would be only a month or two before I'd have my very own apartment. I would be working the night shift, and it would be quiet enough for sleeping while the rest of them were at work during the day.

The information pooled on my frontal lobe like oil; it would take time to absorb. I could think of only one thing: I was responding to a call that would require far more from me than the brand new Littmann stethoscope and the seven new pairs of scrubs I'd purchased for the occasion.

On my way to the parking lot, contract in hand, I thumbed through a folder of useful information that the nurse recruiter had given me. It included brochures for nearby tourist attractions—the Grand Canyon, Lake Powell, Las Vegas—as well as a single sheet of pink paper that listed essential Navajo phrases. *Ya`at`eeh* (hello). So many letters, strung together in unfamiliar patterns "Ya`at`eeh," I practiced aloud, nearly bumping into a wizened man bent over a cane, whose handle he gripped with both hands. He looked up and gave me a toothless grin, smiling through milky eyes. He said something that sounded like "There you are!" when I opened the door for him. Without thinking, I smiled back and said, "Here I am!"

The adult care unit, my nurse preceptor warned me on my first day, got a lot of social admissions. "Just wait until the Navajo fair is in town," she said. "Everyone will dump their aching grandmas so they can party for the week. This place will be packed." I could plan on sweating bullets and running my ass off for apple juice and aspirin most of the time, she explained, but it wasn't technically all that hard. "I mean, it's not like you're going to be saving lives or anything," she said. But I knew better.

A year earlier, back in nursing school in Iowa, I had been indoctrinated with the many ways to save a life. After eight weeks of arduous classroom learning, we were turned loose in an actual hospital to practice the fine arts of bed-making, sponge-bathing, pill-passing, and gauze-wrapping under the tutelage of an experienced RN. We were to meet Sally Kelly, our clinical preceptor, that morning outside of the nurses' lounge on Five North. Assembled in the hallway, we scanned the sea of navy-blue scrubs, the young and athletic-looking nurses resembling the ones we knew from television, and there stood Sally, waving with her clipboard. An attractive woman in her early sixties with the trademark white nurse's cap perched on her head, she beamed light from another time as she ushered us into the nurse's lounge.

The nurse's cap, she told us later, was something she wasn't willing to give up. She'd just worked too darn hard for it. She wanted to be identified as a nurse, not just someone walking around in her pajamas. And besides, she laughed, it was the only part of the original uniform that still fit after all those years.

Our class of nineteen was an assemblage of motivated students: refugees from the crumbling economy, baristas with bachelor's degrees from Midwestern liberal arts colleges, a mother, a father, a former Peace Corps volunteer, a Chinese immigrant, and one part-time forest fire lookout/housekeeper/waitress/fledgling writer/full-time dreamer—me. Since most of us were transitioning to new careers, Sally wanted to know what had pulled us in the direction of nursing. She started with me, leaving me no time to concoct an answer that was anything but the straight truth. I told a story about how I had volunteered at St. Patrick Hospital in Missoula, Montana. Paired with another volunteer, an efficient, retired woman from the Congregational Church, I shampooed the hair of critically ill and bed-bound patients. I told of a morning when I felt inspired to use a curling iron to create corkscrew curls for a twelve-year-old girl whose thick, glossy, strawberry-blond hair belied her failing liver. I ignored my partner as she stood nearby, tapping the face of her watch.

The girl's mother later hunted me down, finding me as I pushed the squeaky shampoo cart back to the storage closet. Tears streamed down her cheeks. "You have no idea," she said, taking my hand into both of hers and shaking her head back and forth. "You just have no idea how much this means."

When I finished the story, I glanced around at the blank faces of my classmates and added, "I guess, in a nutshell, I want a job where I can feel that way every day."

Sally, looking as if she'd been holding her breath, clutched her hands to her chest, exclaiming, "Yes! Yes! It's a drug! We nurses are hooked on saving lives!" This elicited a few looks from the other students, their blank faces yielding to expressions that were equivalent to groans.

We continued around the table in the nurses' lounge, everyone telling stories while the dregs in the nearly empty coffee pot sizzled away to acrid char. Sally told the story of her first nursing job in Cook County Hospital in Chicago, back in 1964. "This was before Medicaid and Medicare were implemented," she said, "and the bazillion people in Chicago who did not have insurance had to go to Cook County. The hospital was so poor that we made sheets out of diapers, or diapers out of sheets." She said that there were nights when the pediatric ward's paper census said they had forty kids, but in truth there were over a hundred. The nurses just kept pushing cribs closer together to make room for more.

Sally, unflappable in her white cap, expounded on her nursing philosophy as nurses rushed in and out of the lounge, slammed locker doors, flushed the toilet, applied lip-gloss, and gossiped. Finally, she leaned in and with quiet conviction said, "Nursing is a sacred journey. Now, let's go out there and save some lives."

Weeks later, in the middle of a particularly busy morning of changing sodden sheets, lavishing barrier cream on bed sores, and washing feet, Sally called her ducklings to an emergency meeting in the med room. She reported that she'd witnessed two students teaming up for an obese patient's bed bath, one on each side. And she didn't like it one little bit. "That is a human being you are bathing," she asserted. "A precious human, like your mother, not an elephant being scrubbed down at the circus." The students defended themselves; the nurses' aides had told them to do it that way to save time. "I don't care if Jesus Christ in short pants told you to do it that way," Sally said, smiling, "you're on my time." The two students rolled their eyes as Sally and her white cap marched out the room, on to the next opportunity to save a life.

I gave my first injection, a simple Lovenox shot intended for an orthopedic patient, on Sally's watch. I was so nervous after I uncapped the needle of the prefilled syringe that I promptly jabbed it into my left thumb, which was pinching up the flesh of his abdomen. He never even looked up from his newspaper while Sally casually ran back to the med room and brought me another. While this later became a favorite joke, that my first injection as a nurse was given to myself, I was inconsolable at the time. Afterward, addled by sleep deprivation and self-doubt, I told Sally I didn't want to be a nurse. I wanted to leave every flat aspect of Iowa and return to the mountains of Montana. My life as a seasonal forest-fire lookout and vagabond was a life I knew, loved, and was good at. I was a professional dreamer, I told her, and I wanted to be a writer, not a nurse. "You are all of those things," she said, "*and* you're a nurse." The skills would come, Sally guaranteed, and my confidence would grow. "The heart and soul of nursing, the part you can't teach," she promised, "is already in you."

She then leaned in and confessed, juicily, that nursing hadn't been her first career choice either. She'd had dreams of becoming a water-ski performer at Cypress Gardens in Florida, but her mother forced her into nursing school, where she cried every day. At the end of each semester, she packed up, threatening to move home. I shuddered to think that if the cards had played out in her favor, this woman, who seemed to have been born wearing the white cap, would have whiled away her youth by gliding around glorified swamps in sequined outfits, perched atop pyramids of muscular men. Our paths never would have crossed. "We don't choose nursing," she said with conviction; "nursing chooses us."

I had other clinical preceptors during nursing school; highly skilled, adrenaline-fueled nurses who ushered students to ER traumas and code blue emergencies and let them start IVs on patients. I learned valuable lessons from them too. But I preferred Sally. Sally—who delighted in the patients' stories, who exhibited her sharp sense of humor as well as her profound compassion—would never abandon me, as others would, in the middle of a tap-water enema to take a call on her cell phone.

When Sally told stories about her days at Cook County, most students sat at the edges of their chairs, waiting for a gunshot climax, some sort of blood-and-guts punch line. But I relished the story when its culmination wrapped back around and confirmed the central issue: that we needed to listen to and really hear the patients before the sacred work of nursing could begin. The simple act of listening, she told us, was a lifesaving measure. Even in the nascence of my nursing career, it was something I believed with my whole heart.

Perhaps the reason I believed so solidly in the importance of listening was that I had been a patient myself, years earlier, and my own life had been saved by a nurse. I was traveling across Colorado in 2002 with my beloved dog, Bandit, when a patch of black ice spun us toward a dark and dramatic stop against the concrete base of a light post. When the lights came back on, I was in the emergency room of a small community hospital in northeastern Colorado. Nurses whooshed past my bed, driven by beeping sounds, tending to machines, and too blinded by the blinking lights, it seemed, to address for even a moment my bewilderment or my tears.

   Later that night, my assigned nurse came to the ICU and sat on the edge of my bed. She placed her hand on me and asked where I was from and what I was doing driving across Colorado—the kinds of things a truck stop server might want to know, but which no one in the hospital, not even the nurse who had vacuumed the windshield glass out of my hair, had asked. She sat and listened to the unabridged version of my story. I told her that Bandit, my constant companion since I'd rescued him as a puppy in Mexico, had been traveling with me. She told me the sheriff's deputy had taken him to the city pound, and someone would take care of him until I was released. I told her that my car and all my worldly possessions had been smashed to bits. And I told her about my parents, divorced for twenty years and on their way, together, to see me, pick me up, and take me back home. But I kept circling back to Bandit—my dear Bandit with red fur and a white paw—and how I couldn't live without him. The nurse assured me that she would check on him in person. She gave me her word, and that alone lulled me to sleep.

   The next afternoon, I woke to see her standing at my bedside in street clothes, her two-year-old daughter perched on her hip, a heavy purse on her shoulder. "Bandit's fine," she smiled. "We just went to check on him. I think he's too lonely to eat, though."

The toddler clapped her hands and bounced, squealing, "Pup-pee, Pup-peee!"

"I told Bandit that you were okay and promised you would be back for him." That plainclothes nurse, I realized, was a secret agent for the Divine. When she left that day, she took with her the elephant that had been sitting on my chest, making room for the healing to begin. But her image was forever burned into my brain, carved into my heart.

Had I not experienced that separation from Bandit and had the nurse not listened to me so carefully, I may have never known how to save the life of Rose Bia so many years later. It was my first week on the adult care unit in Tuba City. Early one morning I discovered Rose at the edge of her bed, fully dressed with a polyester scarf knotted under her chin, slipping heavy silver and turquoise bracelets on to her spindly arms. I had seen her X-ray, and it hurt me just to watch her. She had been admitted for a fractured pelvis days earlier and required strict bed rest. "No!" I told her, waving my hands. *Stop! Danger!* "No, no, no!"

Her hospital gown was folded on her pillow, and the compression stockings I'd struggled to slide over her calves hung over the foot of the bed like two deflated white serpents. Agitated, she muttered, shouted, and waved her hands while looking out the window. The woman in the next bed looked up from her magazine and translated. "She gotta get back to her sheep. She's been saying it since she got here."

Her sheep had been racing through her mind while she tossed and turned at night; every time I'd gone to check on her, she'd been restless and agitated. Thinking that pain was the culprit, I'd shown her the Wong-Baker pain scale, which depicts degrees of pain as faces: a smiley-face zero at one end, a deeply frowning ten with tears pouring out of its eyes at the other. Each time, she pointed to the face with the tears. Every day she spent away from her sheep—twenty-five miles down the long and red dirt road that threaded across the desert, which she could see from her hospital room window—gnawed away at her. The morphine wasn't touching that unsettling feeling.

Sheep was nowhere to be found on the intake form, which asked for demographic information, a list of prescription drugs, even the date of the last bowel movement. I called her son and asked him to come in for a visit. After conversing with him about the sheep in the comfort of her native tongue, Rose slept comfortably that night.

If listening was truly a lifesaving measure, as Sally had said, then night shift was a prime time for saving lives. The cover of darkness provided safe cover for the truth to emerge. Confessions, words that people didn't even know resided in them, flew like startled bats into the night. People confessed to stealing things, to hurting people, to loving some and hating others. Once, a birdlike, elderly man was admitted for malnourishment. He smiled apologetically for his hoof-like and gnarled toenails when I removed his ill-fitting shoes. After receiving IV fluids and a warm meal, he told me, "My grandkids are on drugs. They steal my food and my money, and I can't get no rest at home."

One woman with the longest, most snow-white hair I'd ever seen lay with her back to me, telling me that her son-in-law had raped all of her teenage granddaughters, one by one, under her own roof while she slept one night. I sat, crying in silence, wordlessly brushing her hair, each stroke a prayer for her, for each of the girls.

And then there was Jamie, a young man who came to the unit from the ER, having been beaten within an inch of his life by two of his cousins. Each kick to the head had been retribution for some mysterious crime he had committed against his clan—a system of justice that can be understood only by those capable of navigating the darkly woven depths of long-standing family feuds. "They only stopped because they thought they'd killed me," he said.

His Navajo name translated to Sky Blue, he told me. I was sorting through his personal belongings, cataloging them on the pink Patient Belongings sheet in the admission packet: "Marlboro cigarettes—3; orange Bic lighter; Subway gift card; small plastic bag of unknown; powdery contents."

"Corn Pollen," he said, reading my mind and looking sideways at me through his good eye. "It's for prayers." I wrote this down and sealed up the items in the plastic bag along with his bloodstained T-shirt and Levi's.

He needed prayers. The purple-and-red half-moon imprint on his swollen left cheek was the exact shape of a boot heel, and his forehead had the appearance of raw hamburger. The X-ray revealed facial bones veined with fine fractures, like cracks in a windshield. "I will pray for you," I told him, using a hemostat to gently pack saline-soaked gauze into a gash where his eyebrow once was. I wasn't sure I knew how I should pray, or to whom, but I meant it. He parted his swollen, purple lips just enough that I could see the beautiful whiteness of his unbroken teeth and the faintest suggestion of a smile.

The heaviness of these confessions, these unedited glimpses into human pain, would threaten to collapse me into a heap at the shift clock. I walked home, some mornings, and my body took the daylight hitting my eyes as a cue to stay awake and process the contents of my mind. Those were the days when it all seemed to fall apart. I had no life outside of work and no home beyond the inflatable mattress in the nurses' condo where I tossed and turned, squeezing my eyes shut against the slivers of daylight that shone through the gap in the dark curtains. Bandit, my companion through it all, was almost fourteen years old. He was tired and decrepit, like so many of my patients. Content with just a short walk each morning and scratches behind the ears as he lay next to me, he remained a good listener through it all, infinitely patient, infinitely wise.

Discouraged, I wrote to Sally about how I'd come to Tuba City shiny and scrubbed, ready to make a difference. I'd wanted to roll up my sleeves and "clean house," to make things better like she'd done at Cook County; but I was defeated. I was defeated by the administration, the nepotism, the corruption, the impossible work schedule, and the sorrow of the patients. Despite the hospital administration's promise that I would receive my own housing, I was still sleeping at the nurses' crash pad four months later. I was deflated by the hopelessness of it all.

"Oh my dear little one," she wrote back, "I am so sorry to hear your plight, though I am not totally surprised. Funny, it is the exact experience I had when I first graduated and went to Cook County . . . but I still look back on it as the best career choice I could have made. Don't forget, no other professional gets to walk with people during the most stressful, joyous, fearful, blessed times of their lives." Knowing that I loved to hear the patients' stories, she emphasized that it was in that act of listening that I would find my reward—that alone would give me the incentive to make a difference and save lives. Listening had saved her from burning out. She knew that her patients were precious and that she had sacred work to do.

By abandoning her dream of waterskiing at Cypress Gardens, Sally had waded deep into the trenches of inner-city Chicago nursing. And somewhere in those echoing hallways, in the dead center of some desperate night, her life had been forever changed. My own life was changing, too, in that small hospital on the Navajo reservation, where the wind blew sand into heavy red drifts and beat loneliness against the windowpanes, where each and every day presented an opportunity to save a life. And so my own sacred work continued.

Despite the hardships, nursing on the reservation often gave me reasons to smile, even laugh. One night, I reported for duty to discover that the call-light system had been disabled after a burning plastic smell had tipped off the dayshift nurses to a smoldering electrical fire. The fire safely extinguished, we unearthed a cardboard box of silver bells, the kind a short-order cook might slam while shouting, "Order up!" Explaining the proper use of the bells might have been a chore in any milieu; trying to explain it to elderly Navajo patients who spoke only a handful of English words presented an altogether different challenge, even with the help of a Navajo translator. One patient, Leda Begay, only smiled and cupped the shiny bell in her two hands as if I had given her a gift. Later, I watched from the doorway as she walked to the closet and tucked the bell away with the other items she'd stockpiled during her extended stay: toothbrushes, disposable foam slippers, boxes of tissues, tubes of Chapstick, and dinner rolls.

Later that evening, Leda's gravelly voice cut through the night. "Reshoom?" It came quietly, as a question. Moments later, it was an apologetic plea: "Reshoom." I'd been told that *restroom* was the one English word you could expect the elderly patients to know. Restroom—which often came out sounding like *reshroom* or *rushroom* or, in some cases, the mumbled *reshoom*—was not only a petition for assistance to the bathroom; in some cases, it just meant that something, anything, was needed.

I walked into Leda's room. She lay in bed, her small hand raised above the sheets that covered her head, identifying herself as the caller. I helped her out of bed and guided her to the bathroom. She sat on the toilet, staring blankly. I shut the door and stood on the other side, listening for telltale bathroom sounds. After a few moments of silence, I knocked on the door, opened it, and found her sitting above a toilet bowl of clean water. "*Resh*-oom," she said with her brown eyes turned up to me, emphasizing the first syllable. She wrapped her arms around herself and shivered dramatically. Ahh, *resh*-oom, I nodded in reply. I got her back to bed and walked to the blanket warmer, where I retrieved two blankets that I tucked in tightly around her shoulders, then her feet. She smiled and made a long, musical sigh that was followed by the contented sounds of her body giving in to sleep.

Eventually, the wind blew me back out of Tuba City and onto the road to the next adventure. I never did adopt the nurses' cap of my mentor, my friend and kindred spirit. Instead, I continue to pay daily homage by listening to my patients' stories. Through listening, I save lives from loneliness, indignity, and pain. I save them from mistreatment, from anonymity, from hopelessness. Though the task is often daunting, every minute, as Sally promised, is worth it.

KARLA THEILEN *currently resides in Billings, Montana, where she can see the Beartooth Mountains on a clear day. Her work has been featured on Montana Public Radio and National Public Radio's* Morning Edition *and published in* A Mile in Her Boots: Women Who Work in the Wild.

CAREENING TOWARD REUNION

Nina Gaby

As a psychiatric nurse prepares for her twenty-fifth nursing school reunion, she reflects on her decision to abandon her promising career as an artist, the taboo on hugging patients, and the cultural marginalization of nurses.

> This ain't no party, this ain't no disco, this ain't no foolin' around.
> —Talking Heads, "Life During Wartime"

I. Diet

I am on a diet. Just like when I was facing my fortieth high school reunion, three years ago. There will be no old boyfriends to impress at my twenty-fifth nursing school reunion, but I kind of have a reputation to protect. At thirty-four, I was the third-oldest person in my bachelor's program, one of several nontraditionals in a group of very bright and otherwise age-appropriate young women. I was the wildest, the one with the most energy, and I looked nothing like a nursing student—whatever we were supposed to look like. "She's an artist," people would whisper. "She's old."

When I went in for my first interview with the dean about a university nursing degree (expensive) versus a community college degree (affordable, even on my income as an artist), she immediately signed me up for a university scholarship. Done. "Nursing needs people like you."

· · ·

I bring up the diet for two reasons. The first is to frame this essay so it has more general appeal, some self-deprecating humor to balance the more serious, sadder, sometimes angrier stuff about nursing. Let's be honest: does *anyone* consider attending any kind of reunion without also considering a diet? The second reason is that I am still energetic and irreverent, at sixty-one, still wanting to blast stereotypes, and it's important that I look the part. I still don't look like a nurse. Or better yet, this is what a nurse looks like.

So far, in five days, I have lost 0.5 pounds.

(My long-time archenemy may be at this reunion and, in my mind, still a slim twenty-nine-year-old in an expensive suit.)

II. Bedpans

Loudly stated, at the graduation ceremony for my second bachelor's degree, the one in nursing: "If she wants to throw away a wonderful career as a famous artist so she can clean bedpans, so be it." (By my father. My first degree was a perfectly acceptable bachelor of fine arts, followed by an art school graduation ceremony I didn't bother to attend. I had just completed the hardest two years of my academic life, while evidently ruining everything for my narcissistic father.)

Other things that were said regarding my decision to become a nurse:

"What are you even doing here?" (By one of my first professors, dismayed by the fact that I was wearing a vintage cardigan—mohair, burnt orange—over the blue-striped smock that indicated we were nursing students. The smock, despite having lots of handy pockets and a little slit for our bandage scissors, which to this day I have never used, needed embellishment. No one ever said our cardigans had to be new or white. I took the professor's horror at my wild '80s curls as tinged with anti-Semitic subtext, which I promptly argued about with everyone who would listen. No one agreed, yet the arguing established my reputation as an atypical kind of nurse—a reputation of which I am still protective—although it also got me a B in her course when I obviously deserved an A, thereby ruining my chance at summa cum laude, which I also felt I deserved.)

"You are the last person I could ever see being a nurse." (By everybody, especially those who knew I couldn't add a single column of figures and were reasonably concerned by the idea that I might ever try to perform med conversions.)

"What?" (Again, by everybody.)

"You aren't a *nurse*. You're an *artist*." (By old friends who really liked hanging out with an artist, not so much with a nurse. On the first day of nursing school, a new friend quoted a passage from Florence Nightingale's *Notes on Nursing* where Florence, the most famous nurse ever, uses the word *art* to describe how a nurse governs by "the laws of life and death." These laws, she explains, "require learning by experience and careful inquiry, just as much as any other art.")

I remember meeting Dr. (as in, doctor of *nursing*) Loretta "Lee" Ford, the architect of the Unification Model of Nursing, for the first time. She had a well-practiced response for anyone who, like my father, dismissed nursing as nothing more than bedpan-emptying: "So, what is the four-letter word for the contents of that bedpan? Hmm? *D-A-T-A*! That's what it is. It's *DATA*!" Her statement reframed the world for me.

I used a bedpan just once, when I was in nursing school. I was ordered to place it, upside down, under the butt of a woman being prepped for an emergency Cesarean so I could more easily locate her urethra for stat catheterization. It didn't help that I knew the woman from high school— awkward—or that I had never done even a non-stat catheterization, making it doubly awkward. I haven't used a bedpan since. Nor have I cathed a female, for that matter. I went on to specialize in psychiatry but not because of the bedpan thing. Maybe it was about being an artist. Or fashion choices. Most likely it was about individuality and autonomy.

III. Being an Artist

I was coming to grips with that. It was the early 80's, the time of Jean-Michel Basquiat and all sorts of beautiful mayhem. I wasn't a Peter Voulkos, with his huge, raw, masculine clay canvases, or a Rudy Staffel, who managed to do things I would never do in our shared medium of porcelain. I was feminine, small, literal. My work was small, fearful, and beautiful (and sold well). I met Rudy at an invitational show at the Smithsonian, where we were both exhibiting along with other icons of the clay world. Groupies thronged around him: young art students, as well as younger, less-established artists like me. I had no throng, myself, save for my parents and a friend who came down to DC with us for the opening of the show. My father was never happier and made a big party of the event. I, on the other hand, felt displaced, discontent. This was my highest moment, and I did not trust that I could take it any further. I yearned for a voice that I just didn't seem to have.

When I finally realized that abstract expressionism—the artistic genre I had fallen in love with as a child and that, to me, *defined* art—was never to be my forte, I guess I figured I would try something that made more sense. Something better suited to my deliberate and somewhat obsessive-compulsive work style. Nursing occurred to me suddenly, out of nowhere. Not only would I make a decent living and have someone else paying for my health insurance, but my radical feminist side thought maybe I could do society some good by becoming a midwife and performing safe, cheap, covert abortions in my basement, if it ever came to that. After viewing my fifth emergency C-section during my ill-fated Ob-gyn rotation, I realized that nurse-midwifery was about as much an option for me as was abstract expressionism. People quipped that I could make sculptures of bedpans out of porcelain. Seriously? I went into psych.

Little did I know the level of abstract expressionism awaiting me.

• • •

IV. Psych

We didn't wear uniforms in psych. The caps were long gone by this time. The nurses I knew at the university wore suits and heels that clicked along the hallways; some who possessed clinical doctorates wore white coats over their suits and slung jaunty stethoscopes around their necks. I will always be grateful for them, for their modern vision. But there was one, a large black woman, who still wore her cap. This was twenty-five years ago, and she was one of the few black nurses at our hospital. I remember mentioning her while talking about my new life with my mother, who was far less conflicted about it (for reasons that would make another essay) than was my father. My mother understood the patriarchal origins of the nursing cap, but she looked at it differently. She saw it as something special, like the starched white uniforms she remembered from her childhood, like the scene in the movie *Atonement* where the nurses swish by the camera in crisp lockstep. No one in the nursing administration at that modern university hospital could convince the woman to take off her cap. "I worked too hard for this," I imagined her saying in her Southern accent.

I wish we could have it both ways.

In psych, we are like the EMTs of the psyche. Instead of having strangers' blood on my hands, I have their cerebrospinal fluid bathing my subconscious. Over the years, I have worked as a staff nurse in acute inpatient psych, as an evaluator in the emergency department, as a therapist, as an instructor, as the coordinator of a dual-diagnosis program, in private practice, on crisis teams, and now as a nurse practitioner with my own script pad. I have had to keep people alive against their wills. I have had to take away their elixirs and replace them with side effects. I have had to let boards of education know that nurses and doctors in my care weren't following their treatment plans, and their licenses and livelihoods would remain suspended. I have sat with psychosis and hoped for any extant, still-viable parts of people who have tried to do away with themselves.

• • •

Shining a flashlight on the white spaces, the black spaces, the inkblots of all the overheard and underappreciated stories, we in psych sit with the stories of pain and secrets. Yes, there are moments of love too. "Thank you for saving my life." We can talk about love later. Holding out my hand at the brink, I guess I did save a life or two. Twenty-five years.

Who does this kind of thing? This psych stuff? I tell my students that we nurses use psych skills all the time, no matter what our specialty. But what is the net effect on the person who really does psych all the time? Whereas my old clients had deliberated over the celadon glaze versus the zinc white, my current clients have deliberated whether to keep their contract with me to not jump again, whether to let the Greyhound barreling down the thruway pass them by, whether to turn down that crack pipe, or whether to move out of that abusive household. Sometimes, we just sit. Over time, uncomfortable silence becomes bearable. I have sometimes listened to the intense jumble of gibberish also known as word salad. Salad? *Hey, this ain't no picnic,* I say to myself. *This ain't no foolin' around.* The cumulative effect of all these years is that I usually know what people are talking about, even when they don't make sense to themselves. It doesn't scare me a bit. It's just little spurts of dopamine bouncing around and not getting sucked back in fast enough—an intercellular ping-pong game, and I'm just a cheerleader on standby. As a result, I have fewer friends because it is sometimes just too hard to listen to stuff of lesser consequence. My idea of a good time is sitting quietly with my own thoughts and not making eye contact with anyone. I need to be alone so I don't soak up so much that I saturate. My subconscious is usually OK; it doesn't give me a lot of obvious trouble. Once in a while, after a particularly busy day, I wake abruptly at night, hearing my name being called out, worried that I have forgotten to do something for someone. The other night, the cats were howling. I turned over and convinced myself to go back to sleep because they weren't my patients. That's about as weird as it gets.

• • •

We deal with cruel inconsistencies, in psych, that other professions don't have to deal with. When we've done a good job with someone in therapy, we get "fired." Our job is to make them be done with us. Or when someone starts to look really good after a depressive episode, we applaud for a few seconds and then begin to worry whether they are getting better or becoming pathologically manic. When someone really likes us, we might have to consider a whole new diagnosis: maybe they are borderline, or a sociopath. I remember my colleagues in the hospital, the peds nurses, who sometimes took the chronic kids home with them for a weekend. In psych, even a handshake threatens to indicate a boundary violation. One of my best friends during my days as an artist, a photographer who hand-tinted her portraits, told me, "I have to fall in love with each of my models as I work. It's part of my process. Then I can get their lips and their eyes just right." Soon thereafter, in my new world, I would have to draw a hard, dark line through the word *love*, as if a most basic human emotion needed to be censored. And I understand why. My compassion might be my patient's undoing. If I care too much, my decisions might be clouded. And this is life and death.

But how do we decide? I recall my first year after grad school, working as a clinical nurse specialist (CNS) in the outpatient department where all the therapists had clinical supervision as a group. One day, the facilitator was a highly respected forensic psychiatrist who demanded a show of hands—had any of us ever hugged a patient? No one moved. My old archenemy? The one in the expensive suit? If I recall correctly, not even a blink. No one even dared to look at my little hand as it went up, then slowly dropped, defeated, into my lap. I was certain that my honesty would be punished. I imagined I would be fired. I had no idea how I would justify the horrible act of hugging a patient.

The first time I decided to hug a patient was in my private practice. I had been well schooled, as an inpatient staff nurse, that any touch required either a latex glove or an incident report. I sat in my sunny office with a young woman who was not at all psychiatrically ill but who was recovering after her diagnosed terminal illness had gone into complete remission.

During our supportive therapy sessions, it became clear that the most salient issue in her life, what eventually explained her failure to regain her emotional functioning as quickly as her medical team had hoped, was the death of her mother when she was young, a complicated issue that she had never grieved. Until that afternoon, she had worked hard to deny that this was even an issue. One little question that I can't remember opened up the floodgates, like a movie. It sounds simplistic now, but it was a dilemma for me, then. All she needed, at that moment, was to be a scared kid; she needed to be held, but that sure wasn't in any of my textbooks or in the scope of my nursing practice guidelines. I grappled for a moment with intuition: if this was a piece of art, where would I put the next mark? I moved over to the stool in front of her chair and took her into my arms, where she sobbed for the remainder of the session. Within a month, she decided she'd move to Boston and go to grad school, and I didn't expect to hear from her again.

Abstract expressionism at its best, I now always say about psych. Science is the template, but intuition guides the art. And this is art. And, as a quick sidebar, I hug everybody now. Not once has it been a problem.

V. The Serious, Angry, Sad Stuff
(Brief Rant, Which Should Be Worth a Pound or Two)
Nurses help people and are the essential juice behind healthcare, but I worry we haven't made much of a dent. We are still a profession of women, mostly, and we have barely been consulted about healthcare reform—at least, not in the major media—and that pisses me off. I'm sick of hearing what Dr. Drew, Dr. Oz, the CBS guy, or some celebrity surgeon has to say. They themselves are part of the problem. How do they get to define healthcare? Do any of them really need to make so much money? Does the economy of change really have to accept the status quo: pills that cost twenty-eight dollars apiece, surgeons who have to make a million a year? If the surgeons budgeted better, I think they could have paid back

those pesky little loans already. And if Big Pharma hadn't decided that its administrators needed such obscene salaries, profits could be disbursed in a reasonable fashion and meds could be affordable. Loans and competitive salaries—that's always the excuse. Who decided all this? Then we allowed the insurance companies to put their evil little hands into the pot, and we careened out of control.

That we are women is still a huge part of the problem. We let things go because we are too careful or too busy. We could write more letters and show up at more legislative sessions, but we really are too busy. It was hard enough for me to bring up a child in the midst of my busy career moves, even with a hardworking and supportive spouse, great day care, and control over my own schedule. How about our colleagues with inflexible shifts, the single moms who deal with the insults of mandatory overtime and one-dollar-an-hour on-call status? Who take orders from overworked and overloaded people who know even less than they do? Who must negotiate with healthcare decisions that are driven by power, greed, and fear of litigation? The nurses who deal with all this might be better off wearing caps in some patriarchal system that would at least take care of them.

We could yell more, but we would first have to be really sure of what we are saying. And from what I've seen lately, no one's very sure about anything. Look at the pushback, right now, from physicians who don't think that nurses who obtain their doctorates should be called doctors. Instead of welcoming more highly qualified individuals into the mess, they argue about what they should be called? But this isn't about us and them. This is about us.

Maybe it was unrealistic to accept what I was taught by the incredible (well, mostly incredible) professors and mentors I had twenty-five years ago. Or maybe it was just twenty-five years ago. Anything was possible, then. There were role models getting attention. Hillary checked in with us. There were TV shows with strong nurses. Then again, by the mid-90s, both Carol Hathaway and Abby Lockhart on *ER* had decided to become doctors while I shouted at the TV: "No, no, it would be so much better for you politically to become nurse practitioners!" They didn't listen, and Nurse Hathaway left the show to marry George Clooney, anyway. The popular, Emmy Award–winning medical drama *Nurse* had already been taken off the air by 1983 because, Michael Learned said, she "offended somebody at CBS." How's that for art imitating life? Now we have Nurse Jackie, whom we aren't supposed to like—but isn't she hilarious? She sure doesn't keep her mouth shut. She knows more than most everyone else, and for that she should be revered. So she has a little pill problem and sleeps with the pharmacy guy to get her oxys—at least she has a personality. At least a TV show has the word *nurse* in its title.

Why aren't we ruling the healthcare system? There are almost three million of us. Without us, University of Michigan researcher Beatrice Kalisch has warned, there would be "death, mayhem, chaos." With us, anything should be possible. We have a trendy phrase for complacency and avoidance: *compassion fatigue*. Sick and tired of caring.

I once wrote a proposal for an anthology about this crisis, even before the disappointments of Obamacare, called *What Would Florence Do?* I had a publisher willing to look at it. I wanted to send out a call for submissions to all nurses, to get their opinions, and to cull the best-written ideas into a book of essays. I couldn't get anyone to help me out with it. There you go. Busy, burnt out; or shall we call it fatigue? Anybody reading this today want to take a crack at it?

VI. In Retrospect

Much has changed since graduation. I put away all my studio clothes and work boots. Until I moved to a very rural area, I'd never worn jeans to work. It was unheard of. But where I live now, I sometimes do, although it still seems wrong. Like my role models, I usually opt for stylish footwear. A mohair cardigan would still be out of place but for very different reasons.

· · ·

Legally, as a nurse, I will never be able to walk over someone dying in the street, no matter how much I might dislike them. I also try very hard to never say, "How does that make you feel?" I try not to provide therapy for strangers in the grocery line. I am judicious with my eye contact.

I still approach every problem with the nursing process I learned twenty-five years ago. I can't help it. APIE. Assess. Plan. Intervene. Evaluate. I thought it was so stupid, that first day of class. A pie? Really?

I will never again see blood splattered on a movie screen without thinking, *Universal precautions! Infectious disease! Hep C! HIV!* Nor will I ever be able to just enjoy a character study, be it on TV or in written word, without diagnosing the person and deciding that the behaviors are completely implausible, thus ruining it for myself. The same goes for personal relationships. And familial ones.

Psych. I took a break. For a while, it physically hurt to sit all day at attention, making unfaltering eye contact, holding my usually expressive face in neutral. My neck hurt; my arm was numb. The physical pain made me leave the profession. Or was I kidding myself? Physical pain? Hmm. See, every move is suspect. The economy (I needed a job), a good acupuncturist, and a chiropractor helped me back. I am forever grateful. Fatigue aside, this is honorable stuff.

Now, if I could just focus on the easier things. Whom should I hug? What should I wear to my reunion? Does the event justify a new pair of shoes? Nutrisystem or Weight Watchers? If I'd been another kind of nurse, running around all day, I wouldn't have so much trouble losing weight. I'm only sixty-one. Should I just respecialize? Get my doctorate? Take a painting class?

Addendum: December 2011

So, let's just say that I'm glad I didn't invest in a new pair of shoes. And that diet? Two pounds total. Except for the very minor health benefits, the loss was negligible. It seemed as if no one under the age of seventy-two (class of

'61) attended the reunion. And while I am sure there were some great stories in that bunch, no one shared any of them with me. No one from my class showed up. Only about twenty people attended the important lecture by the big deal alum, now doing research at Columbia. A couple student types were in the auditorium. No dean, one retired professor. No enemies.

The poorly attended lecture sounded like the same stuff we talked about back in '86. And I bet the ladies from the class of '61 in their Alfred Dunner double-knits talked about the same stuff too. With so little going on in my department, I ended up attending lectures at the School of Medicine and Dentistry that were standing room only. Bill Clinton was the keynote speaker, and I got to shake his hand, twice. A couple of lost pounds made that feel a little more exciting, as he looked deeply into my eyes—or so I'd like to think.

The woman from Columbia knew her stuff. She had numbers and statistics and quoted the Robert Wood Johnson Foundation and the Future of Nursing: Campaign for Action. Basically, we nurses need to be fully accountable partners in transforming the healthcare needs of the nation—just like we said twenty-five years ago, like the class of '61 said fifty years ago. We talked about how there are too few nurses on boards of directors, not because of a lack of status or public trust but because of a lack of money. We don't make enough to be important.

I hope that afternoon was not a prophecy of a continuing ennui, fatigue, or worse.

Maybe just a bad day, a busy Friday.

And diets, no matter how successful, have a way of reversing themselves relatively quickly. I gained the two pounds back at the luncheons and went home, sad not to have shared the future with the exciting women from my past. But I did find out that Loretta Ford, still alive and able to appreciate it, had just been inducted into the Women's Hall of Fame this past fall, joining nurses Clara Barton and Lillian and Florence Wald. I did not find this out from any colleagues at the reunion but from a friend who is on the board. She's not a nurse. She's a lawyer but nonetheless excited.

In the midst of all this, in unrelated synchrony, the young woman I had hugged in my sunny office so long ago, the one whom I never expected to hear from again, sent me a Facebook friend request. I cannot wait to send her this essay and see how she remembers it.

Addendum to the Addendum: January 2012

She remembers it quite differently. And she became a nurse practitioner.

NINA GABY *is a writer, visual artist, and advanced practice nurse who specializes in addiction and psychiatry. Her essays, fiction, prose poetry, and articles have been published in anthologies and magazines, and her artwork is in various collections, including the Smithsonian's. In addition to a master's degree in psych-mental health nursing, She holds bachelor's degrees in fine arts and nursing and has taught at several universities.*

NURSE NORA
AT NINETEEN

Nora Casper

A nursing student has a mental image of the capable professional she hopes to become someday. But her expectations, as well as her training, are challenged by the firsthand experience she acquires in a nursing home.

M y first patient was a rubber dummy in khakis and a flannel shirt. "I know it's hard to talk to him like a real person," my clinical instructor told a group of us, "but you have to pretend." He had a large wound on his upper right thigh. Apparently, there had been a boating accident. When we asked him questions about his pain, my clinical instructor, a small woman with an intimidating stance and a kind face, answered with her best impression of a deep, manly voice.

"Sir, we're going to take your pants off now to examine the wound," I told him.

"OK, but I have to warn you— I'm not wearing any underwear today," she muttered for dramatic effect. We all giggled.

Our instructor carefully removed the khakis, avoiding the deep gash; she waited a moment before prompting us. "Imagine if it were you," she said. I had no idea what she wanted until one of my peers jumped in.

"I'm going to grab a sheet to cover you up," she announced.

If this was nursing at its most basic level, I was already struggling. There is no way to memorize how to take care of someone. What once seemed instinctual to most of us becomes overwhelmed by technicalities and anxiety.

• • •

A few weeks after taking care of the dummy, we transitioned into a nursing home. A nursing student's first day in a clinical setting is liberating; most of us have waited years to be of actual service to someone. Before we had the skill to take a blood pressure, we filled the gaps by volunteering at healthcare facilities, making photocopies and greeting patients. We tended to our friends by supplying bandages on the go or by holding back their hair when they were drunk and vomiting. We educated our peers on the importance of contraception and tried to "make a difference" in third-world countries during summers and spring breaks. For a time, this felt like real nursing. But the lack of real knowledge eventually made the work more frustrating than rewarding.

I had acquired the skills to perform fundamentals in a few weeks, and the possibility of taking a real pulse, pricking a finger, or giving a bed bath was as daunting as it was exciting. I had earned the right to wear scrubs with my name embroidered in white letters and to offer real help to a staff of healthcare professionals.

When my scrubs arrived, that summer, I tore the package open and promptly modeled for friends and family. I didn't know how to use a stethoscope, yet, but I placed it around my neck for added effect. The scrubs made my declared major a reality. I had created an image of myself as a nurse—someone in between a *Grey's Anatomy* character and the kind women at the pediatrician's office. It was even more perfect in costume. The pressures and expectations of being a student were not part of that image; it was as if simply by looking like a nurse, I would suddenly know how to be one.

In the beginning, we observed as a pack, unsure what to do with our hands. We smiled at patients as they rolled by in wheelchairs; we mumbled our greetings to the staff. We looked at one another when questions were directed to the group, and each waited for someone else to speak first. Our clinical instructor greeted patients without pause, introducing the group of six girls behind her as nursing students eager to meet them. She asked patients about their pain, about the uneaten food on their plates, about their families.

Learning how to be a nurse has always seemed like a distant pursuit, one that is achieved over the course of a lifetime, not half a semester. As a student, I was reminded of the ignorance I had felt as a volunteer who shuffled between patients' rooms. I still needed to ask someone for help with nearly everything, and our roles were unclear to the staff, who were always unsure how to use us. We wouldn't know what to do when a patient gasped for air, or asked us for a dressing change, or needed a tube feeding.

Determining my responsibility in this environment proved difficult. I was supposed to know and practice a set of skills and to show that I was capable of working with others. Aside from those requirements, I was free to aimlessly wander the halls or take on assignments beyond my capacity. I was free to make mistakes without the accountability faced by a real caretaker. The liberty, although in some ways a comfort, was also unsettling.

My fear of being clinically incompetent—of pricking the wrong part of a patient's finger or not hearing breath sounds—disappeared quickly. Someday those fears would be legitimate, but for the time being, I had the privilege to worry only about talking to patients. I could deliver ice water or feed them dinner if lifting a fork was too difficult. I could apologize for the taste of the applesauce and praise them for eating it anyway. I could help the overworked nursing assistants change patients in bed, and when they didn't have the time, I could be the one to ask the patient, "Are you doing OK?" The simplicity of the question often settled nerves. It was also a trigger for a discussion of how the person felt in general; maybe she wanted to complain, or maybe he just wanted to talk. Had I been a real nurse, I might not have asked because I might not have had time to listen. But I did have the time, so I paid extra attention and gave patients the opportunity to say what they needed, even if I couldn't fix anything.

Soon I was on my own, knocking on patients' doors and making sure they had their necessities. Postdinner checkups turned into long conversations. "My ex-girlfriend was a redhead," one patient told me. From looking at him, I had assumed he couldn't see me or my hair.

"How are you feeling?" I asked him.

"Chipper!" he said. Half an hour later, I knew all about his cocaine addiction, the stroke that left him in a nursing home, and the children he didn't like to think about because it was too painful. His nursing assistant poked her head in and laughed.

"He doesn't stop talking," she warned us, rolling her eyes. "But he's a sweetheart." By now, a few of the other nursing students had also crowded into his room.

"I have an anatomy question," he told us.

"Uh-oh," I said. "I'm not sure I can answer it, but I'll try."

"Have you heard of the islets of Langerhans?" he asked.

"Yes!" I tried to suppress my enthusiasm, which I feared would give away my relief. "They produce insulin in the pancreas. What was your question?"

"Oh," he said, "I just wanted to see if you knew that. Most people don't."

I'd remembered the fact from an AP biology class that I took in my senior year of high school. The name stuck. "How did you know that?" the other girls whispered to me. I laughed, proud for a brief moment that I sounded so educated. I scribbled down his name and room number for next week so he would know I hadn't forgotten him.

Later that evening, another man flagged me down from his room, asking for help with eating dinner. "I got the shakes," he told me. His tremor made hand-to-mouth action difficult.

"Does someone usually feed you, or do you usually feed yourself?" I asked.

"Depends on the day," he said. He was sitting alone in his bed. The smell of diapers and reheated yams was difficult to ignore. His pureed meal looked like watered-down baby food on a plate, and the nutrition basics I had learned the year before suddenly seemed important.

"How was your dinner?" I asked.

"Terrible," he said. "Just like it is every day."

"Looks good to me," I told him.

"Really? You'd choose to eat this?"

I tried to laugh it off but realized that what I'd said was as insulting as it was untrue. I thought of ways to sneak him a cheesesteak and some ice cream and wondered how bad my punishment would be.

Weeks later, I learned that this same patient was not the reliable source of information he'd seemed; his cognitive status changed frequently, and it was unclear whether this was a result of his age or the quantity of pain meds he'd been prescribed. I wanted to be his advocate, the one who ensured that staff paid attention to his needs, but I only humiliated myself in front of the people who tended to him daily.

"He's playin' you," the charge nurse told me on my last evening there. He had been repeatedly asking for more pain medication, and a few of us had reminded his caretakers that he needed another pill. "He's not due for another couple of hours," she told us. She spoke with the frustration of an elder and the pity of a friend.

I was afraid to cross territorial boundaries, worried that my efforts to help would just get in the way. My clinical instructor warned us that the staff might be self-conscious as well: "The same way you're nervous about being judged, they are too." We knew that the techniques we'd learned in our labs probably wouldn't carry over in the field—gloves might not be worn, hands might not be washed. She taught us to note these errors but also to understand the realities of everyday care.

One particular certified nursing assistant (CNA) with a heavy Middle Eastern accent and a subtle bitterness was anxious around me. She spoke quickly, combining words she wasn't sure how to pronounce, and isolated herself from the other staff. Besides the language barrier, there seemed to be lingering doubts about her clinical proficiency. Other staff would remind her of her responsibilities and shake their heads at me when she turned her back.

In the hierarchy of nursing, I was already a class above her by virtue of my enrollment in a bachelor's degree program. She expected me to leave the room when she changed a woman's diaper, assuming that it was something that a future RN was not supposed to do. In the world of nursing homes, RNs mostly distribute meds and have less time to spend on patient care. But I made myself available, and she came to rely on an extra set of hands, asking me to help her put all her patients to bed.

"One more, Nora? One more?"

"Sure," I told her.

"It's too much, yes? It's too much?"

"No, it's fine," I tried to reassure her.

"OK, two more? Two more?"

"Yes, two more," I said.

"Thank you, Nora. Thank you so much."

Her appreciation meant as much to me as a patient's. She taught me how to change soiled linens and how to lift a patient from a wheelchair onto a bed. She also taught me what not to do: In her haste, she sometimes shoved patients instead of rolling them in bed. And she called everyone Mama—an unprofessional habit that's easy to slip into after a few hours of a sixteen-hour shift.

I came to realize that, contrary to my expectations, students were more of a luxury than an annoyance in an understaffed nursing home. After clinical, we talked as a group about some of the issues at hand—the CNA who asked me to do too much, the RN who thought we were naïve. We discussed our patient who had asked for pain meds.

"Maybe she's right that he's playing you," my clinical instructor told us, "or maybe his nurse had a deaf ear."

This sounded like the case studies we read, but their apparent reality was upsetting. How did we know if his pain was real? How did we know if his nurse knew him well or if she had just stopped listening? More important, when we are the charge nurses giving out meds, less than three years from now, how will we know what to do? Will we suddenly acquire the insight and moral compass that will help us to make decisions?

We considered what the nurse could have done in that situation—what we might have done had we been in her position. We could have comforted the patient by listening or encouraged him to ease the pain with relaxation; maybe we could have talked to the physician and found a better medication. But that discussion is a classroom luxury. In a facility with thirty patients and two RNs on one floor, there is no discussion; there is only moving and running and calling and asking. So we learned to be both critical and practical and to recognize that we might also cut corners, someday, in our efforts to do what's best.

•   •   •

I am entering nursing with the understanding that the job will be a series of sacrifices. I'd like to believe that the ideal—holding patients' hands and reassuring worried families—still exists. I'd like to believe that this ideal is what drives people to pursue nursing. But I also realize, as hospitals get more crowded and healthcare becomes increasingly specialized, that the skill to insert a catheter or distribute meds may be more valuable than my compassion. Even if the most human part of nursing gets lost in protocol and formalities, I am sure that it will not be lost on the patients; the small gestures, however few and far between, are what people hold on to. For now, I can enjoy the long conversations about ex-girlfriends and pancreatic cells and appreciate the patient who remembered my name.

Walking home from clinical on a Wednesday night, I watched as girls stumbled from their dorms in four-inch heels and tiny dresses. For a moment, I felt self-conscious in the scrubs I had been waiting months to wear. They were having fun, and I was worrying about the woman I'd just left, who had complained that her legs were throbbing. But the satisfaction I felt from being there overwhelmed my worries and my insecurities. Nursing students want to feel like normal college students. We sometimes even defend our ordinariness, convincing English and international relations majors that we, too, take "regular classes." But I have come to accept that our education is not comparable to others'. The curiosity of my friends usually lies somewhere between genuine and morbid: "So you actually cleaned up poop?"

Understandably, they cannot relate.

Once in a while, I consider the possibility that I am missing out. If nursing is the series of sacrifices I expect it to be, perhaps I have already started by giving up the traditional four years of college. I wouldn't trade an evening on the floor for any night out.

The ease I feel talking with patients has given me a new confidence. My parents were as anxious about my first clinical as I was; afterward, I called them to eagerly announce that I'd made the right career choice. Outside of the clinical setting, though, I struggle to memorize the functions of anatomical structures and to calculate a standard deviation. There is an academic side to nursing school, too, and when we're not at the bedside, we worry about papers and class projects and GPAs like any other student. Friends and family often assure me that personality, not test scores, defines the best kind of nurse, yet I doubt my capability to be more than a good conversationalist and listener. Can a student with Cs be well educated? I want to be a skilled clinician who demonstrates knowledge as well as empathy.

At the end of my first clinical course, I thanked my clinical instructor for her skill and support. She answered, "You will make a great nurse, I am sure of that." Now I must determine what those qualities are, so I can live up to such a title. A great nurse, always. I'd like nothing more.

NORA CASPER *is a native of Hastings-on-Hudson, New York, and a 2010 graduate of The Masters School in Dobbs Ferry. She is pursuing a bachelor of science in nursing at the University of Pennsylvania.*

FOUR STICKS

Janice Dvorak

A Hodgkin's lymphoma survivor goes on to become an oncology nurse. Now retired, she looks back on her life as a series of "sticks."

I.

I laid my hand, palm down, on the white Formica table, and we all stared at it. The nurse leaned over the doctor's shoulder and squinted. The doctor frowned and tapped what had once been a thick, spongy blue vein but now resembled a knotted lavender string just under my skin.

When I was admitted into the hospital, three months earlier, after coughing for months and almost passing out during tryouts for the high school drill team, a robust Jamaican phlebotomist came to my room. My blood spurted all over the stiff white linens when she stuck me. She yanked the tourniquet off with a deft snap of her fingers, laughing. "You got some great veins, baby girl."

Not anymore, thanks to the chemotherapy for my cancer: Hodgkin's lymphoma.

The doctor thumped a spot higher on the back of my hand and sighed.

"If you didn't keep it so cold in here, my veins might be more dilated," I chided.

He grinned at his nurse, then said to me, "You're learning."

I *was* learning. It was 1977, and doctors were on sky-high pedestals. Patients asked questions, but not too many. Medical records were the exclusive property of the doctor or the hospital. Even my parents, who were not cowed by doctors when it came to their kid, were taken aback when I demanded to read a report. They didn't know that one of my favorite hospital nurses, Cookie, had given me my chart to read one night. This was unheard of at the time, and Cookie must have knowingly risked disciplinary action—if not her job—for me.

Cookie was typical of the nurses who empowered, indulged, and cared for me. After a succession of bad roommates (including the one who regularly informed me, in great gory detail, of someone she'd known who had died from whatever the doctors were currently testing me for), they coded the other bed in the room as occupied, ensuring me a private room for the duration of my stay. They gave my friends surgical tape to put up posters and let groups of them visit despite the two-visitors policy. They danced along to records I played on my portable player, which was probably forbidden.

"I think I can get this one," the doctor said. "It's not too bad." He rubbed an alcohol swab over my hand until the skin shone like wet putty; I was that pale. His tapping left a mottled pattern of fingerprints on my hand, like kisses from a child's small, jam-stained mouth—strawberry now, but the next day they would darken to grape or blackberry.

The doctor held my fingers tightly while he used his other hand to take the needle from the package held open by the nurse. It's called a butterfly because the actual needle is nestled between two flat and green plastic wings that make it easier to grip. He pinched the wings back between his steady fingers, baring the needle's sharp, glinting tooth ready to bite through my skin and deliver the clear, innocent-looking liquid that had ruined every vein in my hands except the one he had chosen. Unless it, too, was ruined.

The nurse handed the syringe and the coiled tubing to the doctor. His thumbnail was buffed as smooth as bone, pink with blood. His pulse beat against my fingers like some intimate, silent alarm clock. Or a countdown. I imagined an ignored child tugging at my sleeve, urging, "Hurry, hurry." If not for the vomiting and the damage to my veins, I'd have sworn that the syringe was filled with cold water. But I knew its contents meant that I might graduate from high school, go to college in Boston, write hit songs, become a published poet, lose my virginity, and maybe even be free of hospitals and doctors for a good long time.

II.

My instructor lounged in the doorway, distant enough to give me some semblance of authority and independence despite my blue, pinafore-like student nurse apron yet close enough to observe my smallest movement and intervene, if necessary. I introduced myself to an elderly man clutching a sheet to his chest. His eyes were bloodshot, cloudy with cataracts; his last documented weight was fifty-seven pounds. He would die in days, if not hours, but he was in pain and had requested Demerol. If I told him that his intramuscular injection would be my first, would he refuse?

He wasn't the only one who could refuse. My slender instructor, Sherry, whose blond, frosted hair was as close to the iconic Farrah cut as you could get away with in 1989 and still be stylish, warned me that his wasted muscles would make this a difficult stick. I should only attempt it if I felt confident. I was a student; I wouldn't have felt confident had he been a three-hundred-pound bodybuilder.

My instructor would check me off once I successfully performed this required skill, and I would be permitted to give injections under the supervision of the floor RNs, who were happy to mentor students who didn't hide from procedures. The fear of messing up and failing the semester's entire clinical section, however, was a real one; one day, we'd begun with eight student nurses and ended with four. But I wanted to get as many sticks under my belt as possible while I still had a nurse hovering nearby, ensuring that I was doing it right and giving me tips. That was my strategy with all procedures and interventions, but being good with a needle was my priority from the moment I'd decided to become a nurse.

Needles have a cumulative effect, and enough bad sticks can leave mental as well as physical scars. I'd been stuck a lot during and since my cancer treatments, and not always successfully once I became a tough stick. Most times, I was prepared for the inevitable hunt, the frequent second stick when the first one failed. But every so often, without warning, I couldn't face the needle; I once even required laughing gas at the dentist's office, surprising both myself and my long-time dentist.

I stepped on the pedal that should have raised the bed. Nothing. It wouldn't crank manually either. The staff nurses had taught me to smear stuck frames with body lotion from the patient admission packages, but the bars on this bed were too bent and dented to move. My only option (I assume Sherry would have at least hinted, had there been another) was to crouch down, my shoulder just clearing the bottom of the sink.

What was I doing? I was never going to give a successful injection. For a second, I thought about bolting down the hall, thick-soled shoes squeaking, out to my car and back to the cushy corporate job I'd left for nursing school.

I struggled with illness for several years after chemotherapy and radiation therapy. Doctors warned me that it would take two years to feel normal, or near-normal, but my immune system remained weak, probably because of the loss of my spleen. I suffered from frequent and severe upper respiratory infections, lasting from weeks to months, and near-fatal bouts of chicken pox and mononucleosis. Once an honor student, I dropped out of college; even when I dragged myself to campus, I often couldn't manage the walk to class and could barely stay awake when I did. I quit a series of jobs before I could be fired for absenteeism, yet my employers recognized that I came to work even when extremely sick and that I was a good worker otherwise.

Finally, I started to feel better and landed a good job with a major corporation. The salary and benefits were generous, and I was promoted faster than was technically allowed. I still got sick easier and stayed sick longer than most people, but I wasn't bumping up against the attendance policy. My supervisor mentored me, promising a management position if I got a college degree, which the company would pay for.

I had started working toward a business degree and was doing well, even after my father was diagnosed with cancer and my older sister, who struggled with health problems resulting from juvenile diabetes, developed kidney failure. I worked nights and weekends so I could spend the days with my father and sister in hospitals and doctors' offices.

Soon I realized that I felt more pride when I found a comfortable position for my pain-wracked father or when I rearranged my sister's apartment so she could reach things from her wheelchair than felt when I caught an error that saved my company millions (although, admittedly, that did result in a nice bonus for me). After watching even the best-intentioned family members of other patients, I also realized that caring for the sick didn't come so naturally to most people. I'd try to anticipate what the nurses might do for my father or sister and was often right. When doctors and nurses relayed medical information, I seemed to understand it faster than anyone else. And it didn't just make sense; it was fascinating.

I quit the corporate job, applied to nursing school, and took a part-time job registering patients in an emergency room. On my first night, the other registrars, nursing students themselves, hauled out every ER horror story they had and threw me into every bloody trauma that came through the door. They sent me to register a frequent flier—a homeless drug addict we saw at least weekly who was known to smell bad enough to make even experienced ER staff gag—without teaching me to first put Vicks VapoRub under my nose. I hadn't been certain whether I could handle the gore, the chaos, the pressure; thanks to their initiation, I knew by the end of the shift that I had found my home.

The ER nurses and (to a lesser extent) the doctors monitored the progress of nursing students. Whenever they could, they pulled us into rooms to demonstrate procedures and show us interesting cases. They knew which skills we would be learning and practicing during each clinical rotation and wanted to know when we had completed them.

I now had a chance to try my first intramuscular injection. I'd like to think that something other than a desire to report my accomplishment to my ER family spurred me on. Whatever it was, I reached between the bed rails and used the patient's too-prominent bones to locate the meager swell of muscle at his hip. I mentally ran through all Sherry had taught us, as well as the pointers from the RNs and LPNs on the floor. If I went too hard, I could hit bone, which I'd been told would affect me more than the patient. Not hard enough, and he would get the pain of the stick without the medication, and we'd have to begin again.

I rubbed his skin with an alcohol swab and let it dry, jabbed, aspirated, and pushed the plunger. I withdrew and rubbed the muscle to disperse the medication. I was out.

The man didn't flinch at any point, but I'm not sure I could take any credit. He may have been too exhausted to move. I wanted to ask if I'd hurt him, but if I had, asking would only make him remember the pain. I helped him to reposition himself and asked if he'd like anything. He relaxed into the Demerol.

As we walked back to the nurses' station, Sherry put her arm around me and said, "Great job. I don't think I could have done that." Her relief was palpable, which meant that her calm demeanor had been an act, just like mine. She knew

I might fail, but she let me try. Still, she wouldn't have exposed a patient to a student who she'd thought had no chance of success. Belatedly, I realized that she had confidence in me, that I'd shown her something in the early weeks of the semester that had convinced her of my ability to handle such a difficult stick. I told myself to remember this while fighting the urge to cut and run from my first complicated dressing change, my first catheterization, my first chest tube. For a few seconds, I felt good, but there was still a long time to go until graduation.

III.

The man's arms were the color of darkly stained wood; they would be almost as resistant as wood to my needle, if I ever found a place to aim it. Long ago he had been burned, and his flesh was ridged and rippled like a windblown desert. It was the middle of the night, and he had awakened to my unfamiliar face. His regular nurse had walked me to the room, but before she could wake him to introduce me and explain my presence, a call bell summoned her down the hall. I touched his shoulder and used his name to reassure him. I told him my name and purpose—I was there to replace his blocked IV.

He sighed. I could have explained that I was from oncology, that nurses on my unit were sometimes called to the other floors (except pediatrics) for the worst sticks, and that the nursing supervisor chose the best from whoever was working. Tonight, that was me. But emphasizing how difficult a stick he was would have only increased his anxiety, so I got on with it.

He dozed off as I poked and peered, but I soon resorted to more aggressive actions that fully roused him. I applied a warm compress, had him dangle his arm to the floor, anything to get as much blood into his arm as possible and make the veins more prominent. My adrenaline was pumping. I had to get the IV in for this patient, as well as for my own. Another nurse was covering for me, but she also had too great a patient load.

When I started that job, the nurse-to-patient ratio was one nurse to four patients, then it increased to six, eight, nine, and sometimes twelve. Triple the patient load in just two years. We knew it was because of budget cuts and indigent care, but we were stretched far too thin. I hadn't had a lunch break in a month, and nurses routinely stayed late, unpaid, to chart. Bathroom breaks were rare, so we chugged cups of cranberry juice at the beginning of shift to help stave off urinary tract infections. (This is not an old wives' tale.) When starting toward a patient's room, I would automatically clamp my hands over my pockets; I didn't want to send hemostats and pens skittering across the floor as I ran. When pulling meds or charting, my fellow nurses and I muttered to each other about moving on to less intense settings—doctors' offices, desk jobs. But we loved bedside care. When we talked about giving notice, it wasn't because of missed breaks or bursting bladders; it was due to the fear that we were giving substandard care. It was the fear that one of our patients was going to die because we were understaffed.

I was lucky to have been hired for a renowned oncology unit when I had only nine months of experience as a floor nurse. Even on the mornings when I left exhausted and angry at the patient load, I could list at least one thing I had learned that made me a better nurse.

I had wanted to be an oncology nurse since I'd decided to become an RN. As a cancer survivor, I hoped I would relate to my patients and better address their needs. It seemed to be working. Other nurses sometimes asked me to visit their patients and reveal that I was fifteen years past treatment. I wondered if that seemed long or short to them. To me, it was both. Long because each year was an accomplishment and took me further away from treatment. Short because I was still waiting for my health to normalize, and because there had been so many advances in only fifteen years: improved medications for treatment and for the management of side effects implanted access ports and chemotherapy administered with free-flowing saline, which dilutes the medication and helps to spare the veins. When I took a course to become certified to administer chemotherapy, an instructor said that nurses had suggested and pushed for these improvements after they took over the task of administering chemo from doctors. I've never been able to verify that claim, but when I think of the nurses who have cared for me or my family, as well as the nurses with whom I've worked, it seems plausible.

Such improvements weren't going to help the burn patient I'd been called to stick. His hands were a mess; no veins there. But at a low point between ridges on his arm, my finger found a sliver of give. It could merely be less-severely burned skin, but it was the only thing that felt remotely like a vein. It was higher up on his arm than I'd have liked; if you miss on a stick, you can go higher on a vein but never lower. His other arm was speckled with misses, most of them new enough to disqualify the vein. From second to second, my mind changed about whether I was going to be successful, but I was like that about all but the easiest sticks. I'd worry if I felt as confident as I pretended to be.

I aimed, and it was good. The man smiled and thanked me, and he was asleep again before I finished taping the IV down. His nurse was leaning over a patient in another room, and I gave her a thumbs-up as I passed. She rolled her eyes skyward, then mouthed an emphatic "Thank you." I shrugged, mouthed back, "Anytime," and ran to the elevator.

IV.

My husband, Greg, nudges me—not because he's noticed me dozing off in my chair, but to show me a toddler bouncing and babbling with delight over a toy train. When we first arrived this morning at the waiting room shared by the children's cancer clinic and the adult survivors of childhood cancer clinic, Greg could barely look into the adjacent play area. But he's starting to see past the bandages and IV tubing and bald heads. He grins and waves to a little girl in a pink bucket hat who is waggling a stuffed bear at him. I'm glad to see him adjust so quickly. There has been little illness in his family, and he is still getting used to hospitals and doctors.

In my early forties, twenty-six years after my last treatment for Hodgkin's lymphoma, I've developed late effects: medical problems caused by the cancer treatments that can take decades to show up. I recently learned I have a form of heart failure called cardiomyopathy, but I also have a long list of symptoms, the causes of which have proven elusive. My primary care physician has sent me to one of the few clinics in the country dedicated to adult survivors of childhood cancer.

Jill, the nurse practitioner, takes my history and decides what specialists I will see. She has short dark hair and a face my mother would describe as "sweet, but not the annoying kind." I relate my symptoms. "I have *such* fatigue," I say. "I have to nap at least twice a day. I really do. I don't want to, but I have to."

Jill puts her hand on mine. "We see that a lot with Hodgkin's survivors."

She reassures me when I bring up other, odder symptoms. The multiple cases of chicken pox, neck weakness, xylophone chest and upper body weakness, memory and cognitive issues. By the time we're done with my history, all the things that have marked me as different, that have made me feel like a freak, are normal. They've seen thousands of long-term Hodgkin's survivors, so they have a profile. I fit it. I fit in. Jill makes sure I know that.

I want to climb into Jill's lab coat pocket and stay there, but she sends me back to the waiting room. I see doctors who know late effects. One after another, they examine me and suggest screenings for damage to my lungs, heart, bones, nerves, muscle, brain, and gut. I take notes, but after a few hours, predictably, my energy flags. I can't remember the meanings of some common medical terms. I flub my history once or twice, which makes me a *poor historian*. As a nurse I dreaded taking histories from patients like me. Each specialist confirms what my primary care physician has said: my symptoms are related to specific and mostly progressive late effects; there is little that can be done.

I tried less physically demanding jobs for several years, leaving my beloved oncology floor for a rehab unit, then for hospice. I began to pass out if I stood longer than a few minutes. I was often sick and, because of muscle atrophy, lacked the upper body strength to move patients. Almost a decade ago, I tried desk nursing, which meant medical case management with no direct patient contact. I envied the field RNs I supervised, but I was still a nurse. Eventually, even that was too much.

It's after five o'clock in the evening by the time I've seen every doctor and am directed to the blood draw area. Our footsteps echo as we pass the empty exam rooms. Greg waits outside. It is one of the only times we've been apart today. The phlebotomist has gone, leaving a student nurse who has apparently been checked off for blood draws to finish up. Her green scrubs are new, white running shoes pristine. As she bends over my arm, a red ringlet escapes her scrunchie, and she blows it back off her face. "Maybe I should call someone," she murmurs.

It's hard to feel whiny when I've seen children under active treatment laughing and playing all day, but my inner toddler is having a full-on tantrum. How can there only be a student nurse to deal with my crappy veins? Nowadays, with implanted access ports and other vein-sparing procedures, she may have never seen a stick as bad as me. I'm exhausted and in pain. This is a premier cancer facility; there must be scads of nurses as good as or better than I ever was, and I get a student. Her demeanor tells me this is unusual, so perhaps someone has been called away or is ill. I remember those days.

I had labs drawn two days ago, and my one good vein and my distant second best were both stuck. That leaves the veins I wouldn't have liked to attempt in my prime.

She knows enough to use a butterfly needle, gentler than a conventional needle (I'll later learn that this is now standard procedure), but she's shaking ever so slightly. She taps invisible veins, moves the tourniquet from arm to arm.

I want to tell her how good I was, that I could get a hard stick like me once—harder, even. I want to say, "I am more than you see. I used to make a difference. I was a nurse and a damned good one."

I say nothing and instead will myself to relax as she taps a tough old vein that no one's gotten in decades. At my best, I'd have tried it only as a last resort. Which is what this is. It's going to hurt and probably for nothing.

"Is this one OK?" Her eyes are huge.

"Sure." I sit back and smile as though she's about to paint my fingernails. It hurts, and she frowns at the resistance, but after an adjustment my blood fills tube after tube. She pops the tourniquet, removes the butterfly, and has me press the gauze she has applied to the puncture site.

I say, "I didn't want to tell you before, but no one's gotten that vein in over twenty years." Her milky cheeks go paler, then she blushes. "You should feel really good."

All day I've been a patient repeating my history, listing my symptoms, watching people do what I want to be doing, aching to be one of them again. Now, for a few minutes with the student nurse, I am, even if I'm the only one who knows it. The patient in me wanted to warn her, to insist that she find someone more experienced. The nurse in me recognized a budding professional and took the opportunity to mentor her as I'd once been mentored.

I've been dreading the arrival of my RN license renewal for months. It's hard to justify spending almost two hundred dollars on something I will never use again, especially now that I no longer earn a salary. Thirteen years ago, my mother called me at my first nursing job to tell me I was an RN. (I'd asked for my nursing board results to be delivered to her house; I worked days, and she was home.) The entire unit—nurses, doctors, aides, assistants, patients—whooped and celebrated with me. All the classes and tuition, all the studying and worrying and practicing came down to that piece of paper. It was my whole career. It was every possibility connected to being a nurse. Earning that license was communal, as were the privileges it conferred. Giving it up, if I could bring myself to do so, would be solitary. Without that piece of paper, I will lose the *registered* part—but I will still be a nurse. As Greg and I head to the elevator, I decide that when the renewal form arrives, I will be able to let it go.

JANICE DVORAK *received an MFA in creative writing from Emerson College. Her work has appeared in* Willow Springs, Superstition Review, *and* The Florida Review. *She lives outside Boston with her husband.*

MESSIAH,
Not Otherwise Specified

Janet Gool

A nurse in a mental health center in Jerusalem tends to several patients who share a common conviction: each believes himself to be the Messiah.

Of the thirty-six Messiahs whom I met at the Kfar Shaul Mental Health Center in Jerusalem, Benjamin was one of the most memorable. The majority of our patients suffered from schizophrenia, but Benjamin had been diagnosed with bipolar disorder. We never saw his depressed state because the doctor at the community clinic was able to manage his treatment; his manic state, however, required the intensive care of the acute admission ward. He would arrive in a blue, gold-embroidered custom robe that combined aspects of the garment worn by the High Priest in the Temple, described in the eighth chapter of Leviticus, with features of the robe worn by the Sephardic Chief Rabbi of Israel. His speech was every bit as outrageous as his costume. The product of Iraqi-Jewish parents who had immigrated to Brooklyn, his Hebrew bore witness to both his heritage and his birthplace.

Benjamin often chose to pray below the focal point of the ward, a wall-mounted television protected by a Plexiglas cage. It was usually tuned to station twenty-four, the Israeli equivalent of MTV. Dressed in his biblical robes, Benjamin appropriated the eight floor tiles directly beneath the television and began to recite traditional morning prayers to a hip-hop tune. Rather than swaying back and forth, as Jews often do during prayer, he jumped, twirled, and danced in the tiny space.

The Colombian-born, half-Lebanese singer Shakira, a favorite of the patients, appeared on the screen. She sang her sultry "Hips Don't Lie" as her body gyrated in a belly dance that was familiar to our Middle Eastern patients.

"Hey, guys! It's Shakira!" one of the patients called. At least thirty patients gathered in front of the television. The janitor parked his mop for a moment and joined them as they admired the lovely and seductive singer.

Benjamin continued his hip-hop prayers. Anywhere else, his lithe dancing body, his penetrating eyes, and his unusual outfit would have captured anyone's attention. In the admission ward, he was merely a distraction.

"Janet," a patient pleaded, "do something about him." He pointed to Benjamin. "We want to watch Shakira."

"You've been praying long enough, Benjamin," I said. "Either stop or find a quiet spot at the end of the hall."

Benjamin moved sheepishly away from his spot and walked down the hall with me. "I can't believe you told me to stop praying," he said, sounding disappointed.

"I can't believe it either," I told him, "but there you are. They'd rather have Shakira." We shook our heads in mutual disbelief.

The Messiah didn't figure much at Mishkan Torah, the conservative synagogue in the small town of Greenbelt, Maryland, where I grew up. Of course we learned Maimonides's "Thirteen Articles of Faith"—the closest thing Judaism has to an official creed—in Sunday school. Maimonides, the twelfth-century Jewish philosopher, physician, and rabbi, as well as the author of *The Guide for the Perplexed*, expressed his belief in the coming of the Messiah in the twelfth of his thirteen articles. Each begins with the Hebrew phrase *Ani Ma'amin*—"I believe."

"I believe with a perfect faith in the coming of the Messiah," Maimonides wrote. "Though he tarries, nevertheless, I will wait every day for his coming."

Nevertheless, none in our community seemed overly perturbed by the wait. Business continued as usual. The Messiah was one of those Jewish traditions, like the commandment against yoking an ox to a donkey, that belonged to a faraway place, a distant time. The Messiah had no more of a place in our suburban town than did a threshing floor.

But our Jewish history class *did* devote an inordinate amount of time to Sabbatai Zevi, the Smyrna-born rabbi who turned the Jewish world upside-down in the seventeenth century. Crowned the Messiah by his sidekick, Nathan of Gaza, Zevi convinced the pious communities of the Levant and Eastern Europe that one could reach salvation only by immersing himself in sin. The Sabbateans, as his followers were known, thus embarked on a voyage of desecrated Sabbaths, unclean food, and wild orgies. By 1666, when Zevi converted to Islam in Istanbul, the entire Jewish world was in shambles.

Why would our seventh-grade Sunday school teacher expose her innocent students to such tales of depravity and destruction? Was the story of Sabbatai Zevi merely a curious, albeit tragic, detour in the history of our people? Or was it a cautionary tale about the dangers of dabbling in Messianism?

The only other times I encountered the Messiah were at Holocaust remembrance ceremonies, which always culminated with the singing of "Ani Ma'amin." Reb Azriel David Fastag, a Modzitzer Hassid, composed the tune in 1942 after being crammed into a train that carried its human cargo toward Treblinka. Despite the inhumane conditions in which he found himself (or perhaps because of them), Reb Azriel's thoughts turned to the coming of the Messiah. He began to sing Maimonides' twelfth article in a haunting, spontaneously created tune. Slowly, the forlorn passengers of the train joined in.

Jews would later shiver naked in the snow outside the gas chambers, singing, "I believe with a perfect faith in the coming of the Messiah" to Reb Azriel's melody. Again, the Messiah evoked images of destruction and horror in my mind.

I left Greenbelt for Brandeis University, then immigrated to Israel, history degree in hand, where I discovered that I lacked the means to earn a living. I enrolled in a three-year RN program at Tel Hashomer Hospital, not far from Tel Aviv. It was an extreme transition: after leaving the hushed stacks of the Brandeis research library, I found myself in a hospital filled with patients calling shrilly for their bedpans to be emptied. But I'm a doctor's daughter. Dad took me on his hospital rounds when I was young and parked me at the nurses' station while he examined his patients. When I turned four, the nurses introduced me to their charting pencils—blue for pulse on the one end, red for temperature on the other—and I drew red and blue pictures that they pinned to the bulletin board next to the resuscitation cart.

Gershom was my first Messiah. The police gently steered him by his elbows since he was unable to see: despite the summer heat, he wore a winter parka, the back of which he'd pulled over his face. I opened the ward's outer doors, ushered the policemen and Gershom into the vestibule, and locked the door behind us. Only then did I open the inner door. This system prevented the patients from escaping.

"A neighbor called us," one of the policemen explained. "He was standing on the roof of his building, near the edge. People pleaded with him to come down, but he didn't respond . . . just swayed a little. We're lucky we were able to reach him."

Gershom sat in the staff room at the big wooden table where we interviewed new admissions. The doctors had crowded the room with a jumble of textbooks, reprints of articles, and advertisements from pharmaceutical companies. I found the confusion distracting, but Gershom, ensconced in his parka, was impervious to his surroundings. He answered none of our questions, swaying in his chair with his parka pulled over his face.

"I think he might not want to look at women," said Dr. Tamar, the medical director. "Maybe we aren't modest enough for him.

"Gershom," she said, addressing him directly, "I am going to leave the room, along with Dr. Svetlana and the nurse. Dr. Boris and Jonathan are the only ones who will stay in the room. All men. So you can take off your coat and talk to them."

Well-known in Jerusalem's professional and cultural circles, Dr. Tamar exuded a refined and sophisticated air that was unusual in brash and boisterous Israel. Patients sensed that Dr. Tamar represented something important and solid. At the end of one interview, a Hassidic patient showed his respect for her by backing out of the room, his body bent slightly at the waist, rather than turning to leave. This is the way a religious Jew takes leave of the *Kotel*—the Wailing Wall—or a great rabbi.

Dr. Tamar had the advantage of a religious upbringing and spoke the language of our Messiahs. She greeted them with a cheerful "Chodesh Tov" at the start of a new Hebrew month and exchanged views with them regarding the weekly Torah portion, which is read in the synagogue during the Sabbath morning service. Her assistants, two psychiatric residents who were smart as whips, had grown up in godless communist Russia, but they'd quickly learned to check the Hebrew date and weekly Torah portion and to express shock at a Messiah who smoked on the Sabbath.

Dr. Tamar had assumed correctly that Gershom was using his parka to protect himself from the sight of women. Left alone in the staff room with the two men, he agreed to show his face and answer a few questions. The men asked him about his referral letter, which mentioned that Gershom had stopped eating and was starving himself.

"I'm not trying to starve myself," said Gershom, indignantly. "I just can't be sure that the food is really kosher. I can't do what I need to do if I eat forbidden or nonkosher food."

"Why were you on the roof?" Dr. Boris asked. "Did you want to jump? Did you think you could fly?" But Gershom wouldn't answer any more questions that day.

Like the majority of the patients in the admission ward, Gershom suffered from schizophrenia, a serious mental illness that warps one's ability to think and function normally. Although schizophrenia has over time been attributed to everything from demons to bad mothering, modern medicine has determined that the disorder results from an imbalance of neurotransmitters, the chemicals responsible for the activity of the brain. Delusions, strongly held beliefs with little basis in reality, are one of its major symptoms.

Schizophrenia is found in approximately 1 percent of the world's population, and the disease strikes men, women, Christians, Jews, Muslims, Buddhists, and atheists equally. While schizophrenia may be an unprejudiced illness, its delusions tend to be rooted strongly in the cultures and values of its victims. At Kfar Shaul, where patients included Jews from European and Middle Eastern backgrounds, Muslims from the Old City of Jerusalem, Bedouin from the desert, Orthodox Christians, and the occasional tourist, we learned a lot about the ways that delusions are shaped by culture.

Patients from the former Soviet Union, members of the mixed multitudes who had made their ways to Israel after the downfall of communism in 1991, often described elaborate delusions involving secret police, KGB agents, and CIA spies.

Arab men often believed their wives were cheating on them.

Jewish men believed they were the Messiah.

Gershom roamed the ward for the first few days, his ever-present parka worn over a pair of sweatpants and a T-shirt; he prayed fervently, rocking back and forth from the waist. He sipped a little water from a plastic cup. He agreed to eat fresh fruit, which he washed carefully to ensure that no "unclean" insects clung to its peel. Only then did he recite the traditional blessing, which ends with "who has given us the fruit of the tree," and nibble the fruit with tiny bites.

Surprisingly, he agreed to take his medication without consulting a rabbi.

First-generation medications, also known as typical antipsychotics, were the only medications available when I began my career in psychiatry. These medications eradicated the auditory hallucinations, fears, and delusions brought on by schizophrenia, yet they also caused visible Parkinson's-like symptoms for the patients. These included stiff gait, tremors in the hands, and in the worst cases, an irreversible side effect called tardive dyskinesia, which can cause patients to incessantly move their lips, stick out their tongues, and exhibit involuntary facial tics.

The new medications, atypical antipsychotics, brought their own set of problems. While they generally cause somewhat less severe symptoms than the older medications, they do affect the endocrine system, and their use can result in weight gain, an appearance of enlarged breasts in men, and diabetes. Like the first generation of medications, however, they eventually stabilize the brain's neurotransmitter levels, allowing the patient to begin remission.

Gershom's remission began approximately a week after he began treatment with Olanzapine, an atypical medication. He was finally able to speak with women in the room. Dr. Tamar, Dr. Svetlana, and I joined Dr. Boris and Jonathan to examine him.

"Do you have a special mission, Gershom?" asked Dr. Tamar. "Some kind of special role?"

Gershom hung his head. "I think I am meant to be the Messiah," he whispered.

"Messiah, the son of David?" asked Dr. Svetlana.

He shook his head no.

"Messiah, the son of Joseph?" asked Dr. Boris.

He shook his head again.

"Messiah, not otherwise specified?" said Jonathan, only half-joking. The doctors moved on, again questioning Gershom about his reluctance to eat.

"I need to make absolutely sure that the food is kosher," he replied. "The Messiah needs to be super scrupulous in his observation of the commandments. That's what it says in the Mishneh Torah: 'The Messiah is learned in Torah and exacting in his observance of all the commandments.'"

The staff nodded. Because of their past experiences with Messiahs, this was one section of the holy texts that they had come to know well.

We had many Messiahs in the admission ward. There was at least one at any given time, and there were sometimes as many as five. After breakfast, the patients and the nursing staff would gather for a ward meeting. We formed a circle of chairs, distributing one nurse for every five or six patients. Most of the patients sat restlessly, looking unkempt and bedraggled despite the best efforts of the nursing assistants. Yellow stains marked their fingers, and they were anxious to finish the meeting and receive their next cigarette.

We felt wary on days when three or four patients proclaimed their messianic roles. Would it result in a fight to determine the real Messiah? Interestingly, the various Messiahs tended to tolerate each other.

"There's room for all of us," one of them once said.

"Where is it written that there is only one Messiah at a time?" another asked. Since no one could quote a chapter and verse to prove him wrong, the admission ward community accepted the presence of multiple Messiahs.

After six months as head nurse of the admission ward, I became accustomed to the Messiahs. Other delusions made less sense to me. I found Arab men's obsession with sexual betrayal hard to understand. Their wives often came to visit wearing *hijabs*, the Muslim head-coverings that cover the neck and ears, and *jilbābs*, cloaks that disguise the outlines of the female body. Sweet-faced, they brought bags with cigarettes, clothing, and homemade baklava. Sometimes they carried an infant or a child in their arms. They looked as remote from adultery as Whistler's mother. One evening, when the patients were asleep, I dared to broach the subject with Achmed, a young Arab nurse. After a few years of living in a rented apartment in Jerusalem and working in Kfar Shaul, Achmed planned to return to his Galilee village and marry an educated, local girl.

"It doesn't make sense," I told him. "How can those men think their wives are cheating on them? They look like poster girls for modesty and loyalty."

"It's a delusion, Janet. It's not supposed to make sense. That's what a delusion is."

Of course, that was what Achmed was taught in nursing school. After years of experience, however, I knew that even if a delusion is a false belief, it comes out of a person's everyday concerns, beliefs, and fears.

"I know that, Achmed, believe me. But a delusion should make sense on some level."

"It makes every bit as much sense as those kids who can't keep their shirttails tucked in or their shoes tied, thinking they're the Messiah come to put the world right."

That made sense. We both sighed. The same thought had crossed both our minds: how can there be peace between Jews and Arabs when even their psychoses seem mutually incomprehensible?

• • •

Unlike Gershom, Shalom needed no prodding to announce his messianic mission. He entered the ward like a heavyweight boxer entering the ring for a prize fight: pumped up, full of energy, extolling his virtues.

"I'm the Messiah. You don't need doctors anymore. I'll heal you all. I'm dissolving the Knesset and sending those bastards home!"

Shalom had lived in the storeroom of a building in a nearby neighborhood, and the other residents of the building, disturbed by his constant yelling, contacted a local social worker. She, in turn, contacted the district psychiatrist, who issued a commitment order. Sixty-three years old and divorced, Shalom was hospitalized in the geropsychiatric ward. I met him soon after I completed my tour of duty in the admission ward and resumed my usual post as the head nurse in geropsych. Shalom was severely overweight; his swollen legs and feet fit only into floppy plastic sandals, and he walked with the assistance of a cane. His black trousers couldn't successfully circumnavigate his girth, so the top of his fly and the button at his waist remained open. He attempted to cover the gap with a large belt. The remainders of hospital meals dotted his white shirt.

The geropsych ward offered Shalom ample opportunities to act as Messiah. He "released the bound," as the Amidah prayer promises, by untying a vest that had prevented a wheelchair-bound woman from falling out of her seat. He relieved a patient who was unable to swallow because of his nasal-gastric tube; he advocated for patients who were uncertain about taking their medications. After all, doesn't the prayer say "sustain the living with kindness," not with tubes and pills?

By the time I met Shalom, the Messiah had moved from the margins of my consciousness to its center. In Jerusalem people talk about the Messiah all the time—in their prayers as well as in ordinary conversation. The Grace After Meals prayer, which observant Jews recite after every meal where they break bread, contains the verse: "May we merit seeing the arrival of the Messiah and the world to come." I had learned that blessing decades earlier in Greenbelt, reciting it many times by rote without paying attention to the passage. The reference to the Messiah now seemed to leap off the page. Of course, I now conducted the daily business of my life in Hebrew rather than English. Once, while gossiping with a friend in Hebrew in the hospital parking lot, the hospital administrator about whom we had been talking suddenly appeared. "Too bad we weren't talking about the Messiah," my friend said. This was not a mere, if novel, twist on the English expression "speak of the devil" but a brief moral lesson: if my friend and I discussed the Torah or good deeds instead of wasting our time with idle gossip, perhaps we would hasten the coming of the Messiah.

During my time at Kfar Shaul, a new version of "Ani Ma'amin" became a hit in the Jewish world. A Chabad Hassid named Avraham Fried recorded the timeless words of Maimonides; but unlike the haunting tune that Reb Azriel wrote on the train to Treblinka, Fried's tune was buoyant and joyful, with a pounding beat. It played everywhere. On station twenty-four, Fried appeared between clips of Shakira and Madonna. People danced to the song at weddings and bar mitzvahs. High school kids and soldiers on leave drove cars with souped-up sound systems through the streets of Tel Aviv, Jerusalem, and Haifa while Fried proclaimed, "I believe with a perfect faith, I believe with a perfect faith." This is the same simple idea that had kept the Jewish people plodding onward despite Pharaoh and Hitler—the idea that the Messiah could arrive on any day, at any time.

Ze'ev was admitted on a Saturday evening after the Sabbath. He belonged to a well-known family in the ultraorthodox community. Early that morning, he'd left his house and marched not to the synagogue but down one of Israel's major highways. Members of his community, worried about Ze'ev's unusual and potentially dangerous behavior, followed in order to protect him. He arrived at the admission ward looking disheveled and confused, dressed in the knee-length black breeches, white silk stockings, and black gabardine coat of his sect. In place of *peyos,* the side locks that frame the faces of Hassidic men, were two jagged tufts of hair.

Dr. Tamar and the rest of the admission staff interviewed him on Sunday afternoon. Dr. Tamar exchanged a few pleasantries before straightforwardly asking, "Are you the Messiah?"

Ze'ev's answer surprised us.

"No, I am not the Messiah. But they think I am."

"What? Could you repeat that? What do you mean?"

Everyone at the staff table leaned forward with bated breath. Here was a novel take on an old story.

"They think I'm the Messiah," Ze'ev said. "The people in my father's community. I told them I'm not. But they wouldn't believe me. I had to convince them that I'm not the Messiah."

"What did you do to convince them?" asked Dr. Svetlana.

"Can't you see?" he said in astonishment. "I chopped off my peyos! Did you ever see a Hassid without peyos before? But they still thought I was the Messiah."

"What makes you think they continued to believe you were the Messiah after you chopped off your peyos?" asked Dr. Boris.

"I decided to get away from there. I needed to get away from all those people who thought I was the Messiah, so I left. I started walking down the highway on Shabbos morning, when everyone should have been in *shul*, in the synagogue, praying and listening to the Torah reading. But instead, they started walking behind me, ready to follow me anywhere. A bunch of Hassids followed me down the highway on a Shabbos morning! Why would they follow me like that if they didn't think I was the Messiah?"

We sat in stunned silence. Ze'ev had beaten us at our own game.

Ze'ev responded well to his medication and became a day patient, visiting the ward two or three times a week for a check on his progress. I greeted him on one of his visits, but he didn't respond.

"Now that you're feeling better," I said to him, "you've returned to the normal behavior of a Hassid. I understand that you're not supposed to talk to a woman."

"No," he said, "I can talk to you. I just can't greet you. It's immodest for a man to greet a married woman."

Ze'ev had artificial peyos attached to the sides of his face—long, straight swatches of hair that reminded me of the tails on toy horses. I wondered where his family had found them. In a costume shop? Had they asked someone who makes wigs for Hassidic women to make them? I didn't ask. It seemed an immodest question.

I admitted many Messiahs in the four years that I worked in the admission ward, but I never discharged one. Gershom, Benjamin, and all the other Messiahs eventually cooperated with their medication regimens and abandoned their notions of being the Messiah, the righteous descendent of King David who would bring about a better life for all mankind. They would not put an end to war or rebuild the Holy Temple in Jerusalem. Suffering from a chronic and recurrent disease that sent them into downward spirals and made everyday tasks difficult, they returned to their realities to study, work, marry, and raise families.

I escorted discharged patients out of the ward, opening the set of double doors. On an outside porch that resembled a truncated loading dock, I handed them their discharge letters, three days worth of medications, and the cigarettes and matches we'd held for them while they were hospitalized.

At first I didn't know what to say when a patient was discharged. "Good-bye" or "shalom" sounded too curt, while "see you again," though honest, seemed pessimistic. I eventually settled on a traditional Jewish formula: "We should only see each other at happy occasions," I told them.

I would watch each patient slide into a car with the wife, father, or brother who had come to pick him up. No, he was not the Messiah, I would think. The real Messiah still tarried. I would stand on the porch a minute longer in the clear, penetrating Jerusalem light, waiting with a perfect faith.

JANET GOOL *lives with her husband, Yochanan, and the youngest of their three children in Beit Shemesh, Israel. This is her first published work.*

ALL ALONE AND AFRAID:
Becoming a Person through Nursing

Anna Gersman

Coordinating home care for an obstinate and insulting patient dying of AIDS, a case manager finds that the patient evokes memories of her abusive father.

I pull into the driveway of my client's home in southern Ontario and park beside an old boat of a car that's covered with a thick layer of snow. One of its tires is deflated, and it's heavily rusted around the doors. I grab my program-issue black vinyl briefcase and give my lipstick and hair a quick check in the rearview mirror. Part of my work as a home care case manager is to immerse myself in all the aspects of my clients' lives—the parts beyond their bodies—that interact with the world: family, home, work, money. I feel like a fraud, a big fake who came out here to do an assessment; the secret parts of my own life are a mess. I scan the chart. "Single man, lives alone. Diagnosis: AIDS. Date of birth: 1929." He's the same age as my father. I block out the twinge of fear and anger that any thought of my father sparks.

I went into nursing for all the wrong reasons. I wanted a job that would provide me with a steady income. I didn't feel kind or considerate, and when the work frightened or repulsed me, I buried those feelings deep down. I hid the neon sign on my head that flashed: Imposter. Liar. Spy. Double agent. A good nurse kept an impenetrable barrier between work and home. I was not real nurse material like my mother and my aunts, Fiona, Nora, and Maureen. All incredibly strong Irish nurses. I worried I'd be like Aunt Una, my mother's younger sister who didn't make it as a nurse. She had a breakdown instead.

• • •

It's a small gray bungalow on a dead-end street. The developers have started thrusting into this area, knocking down the small postwar bungalows and erecting massive monster homes. Generation X wants a library, a pool, a conservatory—a damn Clue game. People with young families like mine have had to move further north, where real estate and taxes are lower. Cautiously, I walk up the icy pavers to the front door. A huge blue juniper overgrows the metal railing.

We are to insist that our clients salt and clear their walkways, according to the highly paid health consultants who periodically attend our meetings; dressed in power suits, they give us advice and community safety tips. "You must tell them they are not eligible for services, otherwise," we are told. "You have the right to work in a safe environment." We'd never visit anyone if we followed their instructions.

Reaching past the claws of the juniper, I ring the cracked doorbell. A broken welcome sign hangs askew on the wooden inside door. Curtains are drawn tight across both front windows. I know from other visits on this street that one is for the living room; the other, smaller one is a bedroom. Scraggly old yews and spiky holly crowd up in front of the windows. I ring again and wait. Finally, after a third ring, I hear a shout from inside.

"OK, OK, I can hear you. I'm coming." The front door is yanked open and a thin, narrow face stares out at me.

"What the hell do you want?" the old man snarls in a thick English accent. He hunches away, squinting behind his glasses as if it has been a while since he has seen the sun.

"I'm Anna from the home care program. Are you Mr. McPhee? I called you yesterday to book a visit. Do you remember?" My heart is pounding despite the cheery smile I have plastered on my face.

"Oh damn, come on in then. I forgot you were coming." He turns from the door, holding on to the wall. I follow him. "Goddamn waste of time. Waste of taxpayers' money," he mutters under his breath. "What the hell is it you want again?" he asks over his shoulder.

Good question, I think. What is it I'm doing? This is a new role for me. It's so very different from hospital nursing, where the rules and boundaries are clearer. It's like going into enemy territory as some kind of quasi-invited guest.

"I have some questions to ask you about how you're managing here at home. See if we can help with something else besides the lady we send to give you a shower."

"If I need more help, I'll call you."

Good point, you old grump, I think. "OK, well, that's great. It's just that I work for the government, and we want to make sure you know all about our services—about home care, I mean."

"OK, OK. Just ask your goddamn questions and be done with it," he says.

The house is shrouded in darkness. A small open concept living and dining room are on the left. It looks like no one has been in there for a long time. The green velvet sofas are old but not worn out, and his recliner sits across from an aged cabinet-style TV. The coffee table is scattered with old newspapers. In the far back corner, there is a wooden dining room set—a retro Scandinavian style from the '60s. Behind the glass doors of the sideboard are shelves filled with dishes and glassware. In the gloom, everything looks coated with sticky, grimy dust.

"Are you from England?" I ask, trying to be friendly.

"No, I'm Irish. Is that one of your questions?" He steadies himself in the darkened hallway, clutching the doorframe of his dim bedroom. "You'll have to come into my bedroom. I'm in bed, most of the time." He falls onto a ramshackle bed. The sheets are a tangled, dirty mess. Crumbs and grit lie in the creases. *Safety orientation: if it's an unfamiliar environment, make sure to sit facing the doorway, always in the living room, never in the kitchen. There are knives in the kitchen.*

"My mother's from Ireland—came over in the '50s," I try.

"Oh yeah. Well, I've been here that long as well."

"Where in Ireland?" I pry just a little more.

"Belfast," he says.

"Oh, Mom's from Clare."

"Oh, the south," he says with a sigh, lying back. His unshaven face is gaunt yellow in the light from the bedside lamp. I drop it, not wanting to touch upon any bitter Irish tensions that might burn just below the surface.

"Do you live alone?" I ask.

"Now what in the hell has that got to do with anything?" he yells, staring at me from behind his dark-framed glasses.

"Well . . . well," I stutter, my mind racing for an answer. "It's just that we need emergency contacts. In case we come to visit and we don't get an answer at the door . . . then we . . . we worry about you. If you've fallen and are lying on the floor . . . so, if there is someone we could call . . . a neighbor, a friend."

He pushes back against the pile of dirty pillows. "Goddamn busybody do-gooder is what you are." He grunts.

"Well, that's one way of looking at it," I laugh. "I'm a nurse, actually. But I work as a case manager now." It feels like talking to Grandpa—cantankerous, critical old shit. He looks terrible. Skin and bone, and dirty. I spent my childhood surrounded by mean-spirited, moody men who felt entitled to abuse everyone around them, insistent that everyone tiptoe around their bad tempers.

"You're a nurse, are you?" He stares hard at me. I wonder if he's thinking, *Some pathetic type of nurse she is.* I really don't know what the hell I'm supposed to be doing.

"Yes," I answer. With a man of this generation, my being a nurse may garner respect.

"Well, there is no contact. I live alone, and I don't know the neighbors, anymore. It's all immigrants now, new people. All the old people have sold or died off. I've lived on this street for forty years, and I don't know anyone anymore."

"OK, well, I have your doctor down as a contact. He's the one who referred you to us for some help."

"Oh, it was him, was it? He's another one. Has to be worried about me, has to keep interfering and trying to help. You people don't think, do you? I have lived on my own for fifty years; do you really think I can't manage without your help?"

"Well, no, Mr. McPhee. It's just that the little bit of help we give people . . . sometimes it prevents a fall and other problems. Are you taking any medication?"

"Now that's another dumb question. You can see all these bottles." He jerks a big hand at his bedside table. "Why do you have to keep asking stupid questions?"

"Can I write down the names of them? Do you know what they are for?"

He stares sullenly at me from sunken eyes, and I want to laugh. He shakes his head. "I'm not even going to answer that." He closes his eyes.

"Do you have a lot of pain? I see you have a lot of pain medication."

"Oh, you noticed that, did you? Well, most of it didn't do a damn bit of good. A complete waste of money. I started on the patch, this week, and that's finally helping me." He sighs. His pillowcase is covered with flakes of skin and smears of blood from sores on his head.

"Are you managing your meals?"

"Yes, yes, I'm fine. How many times do I have to tell you people?"

"Who is doing your shopping?"

"Oh, for God's sake. That woman you sent did some shopping for me." He pauses to draw a breath. "I had a friend helping me before, but he just stole everything. All he was interested in was my money."

I don't tell him that the personal support worker (PSW) should not be helping with the shopping: with the increased demand for home care, it's one of the duties we can no longer fund. Reducing help for this man without family, neighbors, or friends, however, isn't possible. Scanning my long list of questions, I hesitate. The one about his mood is really going to infuriate him. I drop the questions and ask instead if I can look in his fridge and the bathroom where the PSW showers him.

"Go ahead. I don't care," he grunts. The kitchen counters are crowded. An open box of cereal, cans of beans and soup. A drab polyester curtain droops across the window. Below, in the sink, are a pile of dirty dishes, a heavily stained mug, pots, and cutlery. A few bananas wilt brown in a bowl, and a bag of sliced bread sits open near a toaster. The fridge is empty but for a carton of eggs, a package of cheese, some hot dogs, and old bottles of condiments.

The bathroom sink, toilet, and shower are turquoise. The mat and toilet seat cover were white at one time. The sink is caked with a thick ring of scum, and heavy black mold sits in the corners of the shower. The PSW is not supposed to houseclean, and this bathroom is beyond bleach.

"You have food in the fridge," I say.

He rolls his eyes at me. "What did you expect? I'm not dead yet. That woman you send makes me something when she comes in." I tell him she can help with the laundry and wash his bedding, seeing as he's in there all the time. I don't tell him she isn't supposed to cook. He's so thin.

He groans, "Are you done yet?"

"Yes, I'm done. Can I come back and see you again?"

"I guess so, if you have to." He looks ready to doze off.

He reminds me of my father—the kind of man who couldn't show weakness or kindness. This frail, elderly stage must be terrifying. Dad disappeared after the divorce. "You are the cause of all my problems," he'd told us.

"You don't keep in touch with your father?" his sister, my aunt, asked me.

"No," I wanted to shout, "I don't keep in touch with someone who assaulted me and my mother."

Over the next few months, I dread the visits with Mr. McPhee; he continues to be negative and critical. If I pry too deeply or make recommendations, he says, "To hell with everyone. Don't bother, then. I don't need handouts." I don't want him to throw us out and end up like one of those people you read about in the paper—dead in their homes for weeks before anyone notices. He bonds with one PSW in particular. She helps him without asking questions and doesn't insist on giving him a bath if he doesn't want one. She is kind and helps him with shopping, cleaning, and cooking—even if she's not supposed to. I authorize it. Make an exception for him. It's impossible to explain Ministry of Health guidelines to this dying man.

One day, right after Christmas, she calls. "Anna, it's me, Veronica, I be at Mr. McPhee house." She's whispering. I know the peach-colored phone hangs on the kitchen wall.

"Is everything all right?" I ask.

"No, it's not. When I come today, he's covered in poo. The whole bed; he couldn't get to the toilet. He really weak. I cleaned him up good, but he don't want me to tell anyone. He don't want the doctor to know. Can you come and see him? Don't tell him I told you. He be mad. He won't trust me."

"I won't say anything. How long have you been there?" I ask.

"I be here three hours. He won't go to the hospital. I ask him," she whispers. "He weak like a baby, and he eating nothing."

"OK. I'll call your agency and authorize the three hours for today. I'll come see him, but I'll have to call the doctor. Make sure you go in tomorrow. I'll see if I can get him to agree to an increase of your time there."

I call his doctor, Dr. Hill. "Mr. McPhee is having a hard time, starting to be incontinent of stool and urine. He barely accepts any help. He's all alone there. Do you know if he has any family?"

"You know, I think he may have a brother back in Ireland, but I'm not sure. He came in once with a younger man who I thought was his partner, but I don't know. I'm having trouble with his pain management. He's going to need a pain pump soon. What about a commode?" he says.

"I am sending out a commode today and a walker. I just don't think he should be staying there alone anymore. He needs someone to take care of him."

"Well, if he'll agree to hospice. I don't want to force him. I'd rather he made the decision on his own. Do you think he's capable of making decisions?"

"I'm not sure. Last time I saw him, he made sense. He didn't want to leave his house, but he's really at risk, being alone," I say.

"Well, if I have to, I'll get the police to take him to hospice. He'll get good care there."

Mr. McPhee doesn't answer when I phone. I make a visit. The old blue car still sits in the driveway under a mound of snow, tires sunk into the icy pavement. He told me he'd been a carpenter and fixed everything himself—the house, his car.

"Mr. McPhee?" I walk in after one knock. He is a gray shadow lying in the dark bedroom. The house smells musty, like an animal cage. A look of cold terror is in his eyes.

"Oh, it's you," he says, and closes his eyes again. I sit on the old kitchen chair at his bedside, its split vinyl seat poking into my thigh. Used tissues litter the floor.

"Mr. McPhee, I'm really worried about you being here alone. Don't you have a brother? Can I call him? He'll want to know how sick you are."

His eyes fly open. "Don't you dare call my brother."

"I won't call him, but I just think that if you were my brother, I'd want to know what's going on. I'd want to help."

"Well, I don't give a good goddamn what you think. You are not, under any circumstances, to call my brother. Do you understand?" he wheezes from his indented pillow.

"Yes, I understand. I won't go against your wishes, I promise."

"Good. Now, just pull that blanket over me. I'm freezing." After covering him, I sit down again to write out my notes. He keeps dozing off. I tidy his room and sit for a long time, unable to leave him alone in the awful, gloomy stench. A paralyzing sadness builds up inside me, knocking out all objective professionalism. My own pain freezes up my face, burning and choking me.

Over the next week, he deteriorates quickly. His care plan keeps me busy. The PSW does a four-hour shift every morning, but then he's left alone to drag himself to the commode and fill it with diarrhea. She empties it in the evening when she comes back for another two hours to get him ready for bed. His skin gets thinner and thinner; it bruises and tears easily. Sores fill his mouth. Abdominal pain makes him writhe on the bed. His eyes are sunken into a skull stretched over with yellow skin.

Dr. Hill calls on Monday morning. "I was paged over the weekend. He finally agreed to go. I think the pain was just too much. He's in the hospice. You can close the file."

"Thanks for letting me know. Do you think we should have tried to get him in sooner?"

"No, it's hard with men like him. He really didn't want any help," Dr. Hill says.

Cold, hard desolation washes over me as I close that file and shut away his life, his house full of the things he'd carefully collected over years of life and work. He'll be alone in the hospice—no visitors will come. It's cold comfort knowing that he's safe there and no longer my responsibility. A week later I get a call from the Public Trustee's Office. Mr. McPhee is dead. The social worker at the hospice notified them of my involvement with his care.

"He died last night. We have arranged for the funeral. There doesn't seem to be any next of kin except an elderly brother in Ireland."

"Yes. That's right."

"We called the family. They were shocked, of course. Didn't even know he was sick. We have the will—everything goes to the brother. He wanted to be cremated. Do you know of any other wishes he may have had?"

"No, except he didn't want that brother contacted. He was very private and didn't want help."

"The brother's upset, of course; he wants to know why they weren't called. He wants to know what he died of."

"Those were his wishes," I say. "He made it very clear. He did not want him contacted."

"Well, thank you. The funeral will be at 10:00 a.m. tomorrow."

When I hang up, I again feel a terrible rock of despair pound down on me: the sad loneliness of abandonment. The pride I felt for my accomplishment—the little crack I made in his armor so we could feed and clean him—seems pathetic.

"I'd like to go to the funeral of a client of mine," I say to my manager. "He had no family. The Public Guardian's Office isn't going. I think it will only be me." She looks up from a stack of papers on her desk.

"Sure, Anna, go ahead."

It's early on a cold spring morning. The streets are slushy with dirty snow. In a down-and-out area of the city, I find parking behind the small red brick funeral home wedged between tall office blocks. Inside it's silent and dark, the walls paneled with wooden wainscoting. A dark staircase leads upstairs. His name is written on a cardboard sign outside a chapel to the left. Going in, I sit down alone on the cold pew. A plain, closed wooden casket rests at the front of the small room. Bits of light are shining through a small stained-glass window, penetrating the chilled loneliness. I feel defiant, bearing witness to this stranger's stubborn, aloof anger. I wonder if he was afraid to go. He seemed too angry to be afraid. Then I hear him chastising me. *You bloody idiot. Wasting taxpayers' money coming to my funeral. I'm dead; no one cares.* But I argue with him, *I am here, despite what you think and believe and want. I am here as a witness to you. This is what I want. This is for me, you cantankerous old grump.*

My father lay in a casket like this, alone, his past a closed book. He left instructions that we were not to be contacted, but it was provincial law: next of kin must be notified. We were called by the lawyer weeks after the funeral and cremation. Later, his friend called. He knew Dad had been married, but he didn't know there were six adult children. He'd thought he was the son Dad didn't have. I had gone thirty years without speaking to my father. I couldn't bear to call him and have the phone slammed down in my ear, the cold echo of dial tone buzzing and stoking a fire of rage. I was relieved when I learned he was gone but could not—still cannot—let go of my childhood fears of his physical power, his fists and hard leather shoes, his threats and insults.

The funeral director comes in; he is thin, stooped over, serious. I give him a smile, then feel a shudder of false sincerity. I stifle it down.

"Thank you for coming," he says. "I didn't know David McPhee. I never met him. Do you think anyone else will be coming?"

"No."

"They told us he wanted a plain, simple service. Do you want to say a few words?" I shake my head—the right words don't come to me.

ANNA GERSMAN *is fascinated by the power of storytelling—particularly by the stories of nurses. She works as a nurse case manager and writes daily. She lives with her family in Canada.*

INDIVIDUALLY IDENTIFIABLE

Pamela Baker

Nurses draw support from one another by sharing their stories. But to comply with patient confidentiality laws, they must keep silent about things they've seen, as well as the stories patients tell. One nurse struggles with these limitations.

I first breached the confidentiality agreement between myself and a hospitalized patient when I was twenty. This was before the Health Insurance Portability and Accountability Act of 1996—now widely known as HIPAA—and signed a confidentiality agreement, as was then the standard. Such agreements were always accompanied by threats: any divulgence on my part could have led to my termination. I could even have been sued. The offense would have gone on my permanent record, and my prospective nursing career would have dwindled, turning it into a shady, bad idea. But I considered myself a good worker who knew and followed the rules. I wouldn't go blabbermouthing about what or whom I saw—it was a crude idea that conjured up images of ignorant people who liked to tell funny stories at the expense of others.

I was working in a locked adult psychiatric unit when I helped restrain a near-naked woman. The keys I carried made me feel powerful, and I'd bought a special cord for them—a yellow spiral that wrapped around my wrist. I was young enough to feel grandiose in my new position, convinced that my having landed the job was proof of my therapeutic nature; I was ready to transform those in need through my care, to reshape their thoughts of despair into self-assuredness and hope. I had faith that the right words would spill from my mouth, piercing holes in their darkness and letting in light.

One evening I was doing hourly rounds with my clipboard and grid sheet, checking that the right doors were locked, all the patients accounted for. I entered the kitchen, the patients' domain. A woman stood over the kitchen sink, eating cold hotdogs one long link after another, her binge driven by desperation. It was in her care plan to eat less. She wore only a hospital gown for bed, blue angles patterned on white, the back barely tied because of her size. I asked her to please put down the food, the weapon she would hurt herself with. Did she need to talk? Did she *want* to talk? Did she want to leave the kitchen and go someplace else? She smiled in response and stuffed more meat in her mouth.

My position deflated, I left to get the assigned tech—that person's problem, not mine. The tech huffed up from her spot at the nurses' station, as I knew she would, sighed with her eyes, and lunged into the kitchen. "Put the food down," she said. "Put. It. Down."

The tech's tone made the woman stop; she held a bit of rubbery hotdog in her hand as they studied each other, each considering the other's position, each deciding who would give in. An audience gathered as patients grouped together near the tables. I reinforced the primary tech, sharing in her authoritative stance.

"Do you want to do this to yourself?" the tech said, gathering momentum. "You're just hurting yourself. You're not supposed to be doing this. Put the food down. We can talk. You were making progress. You're hurting yourself. Put the food down. Put it down."

The woman threw the bitten pink piece into the sink. I heard it *thunk* against the metal and watched it bounce back out again as she yelled at the tech about being misunderstood. "Why can't you leave me alone? I wish I was dead!" She stomped toward her room.

The tech followed and instead maneuvered her into the seclusion room. Open-door seclusion is a tool that provides the patient with a place to calm down and think about what she has done wrong; if the patient fails to deescalate, the door can be closed and locked for the safety of staff and other patients, a measure that is categorized as a type of restraint. I marveled at the tech's command of the situation and took mental notes of her stance as I watched. *So that's how you handle it*, I thought. *You don't give in. You take control. See it through to the end.*

The woman was now screaming. When she threatened to leave the room, the tech closed the door. "She's out of control," she said.

As she got the seclusion paperwork, I watched the woman through the door's small square window of shatterproof glass as she took off her gown and tied it around her neck. "She's trying to choke herself," I said, attempting to hide the panic in my voice.

Someone unlocked the door. A nurse and one of the techs pulled the gown away. Naked, her smooth breasts sagged, her dimpled thighs shook; her screams were low-pitched and echoed—a white bear without teeth or claws. The door closed, and we were once again on the other side of the concrete and metal, thinking the episode finally over.

"Oh God, she's still trying to strangle herself," the charge nurse said.

Both her hands were at her neck, and her face was turning red. "What do we do?" I asked.

"We'll have to restrain her," someone said.

And we did. As we walked her to her room, I was unnerved by the woman's acquiescent calmness. It didn't feel right. She went straight to the bed and lay facedown, remaining still as we applied the leather restraints to her limbs. Somebody put a bath blanket over her to finally cover her exposed flesh. Tears had replaced the noise, and she eventually calmed completely. She refused to make a verbal contract to stay that way; it was our fault, she said—we should have let her eat in peace.

To get out of seclusion, the patient has to "process out." It's much like letting a child out of a timeout. *Why are you here? What did you do wrong? What are you going to do differently next time?* She wouldn't do it; she came out of the restraints but not her room. She was still there the following day, too stubborn to give in. She wouldn't eat. This was the power she had; the standoff continued for two days.

I felt guilty for my own part in the impasse. I also knew that the patient had passed through the revolving doors of the state hospital many times over the years. When I saw a friend who worked there, I asked if she was familiar with the case. She said she was. "How do you manage her?" I asked.

My friend recalled the patient's stubbornness, how she wouldn't yield to staff when she felt cornered and powerless, how her behavior became compulsive and irrational when she felt she wasn't being heard. It was best to step away from the power struggle, to yield to her a little, and to find a balance where she could be both safe and in more control. Proud of my newfound insight, I shared the information with my coworkers during my next day at work. Shortly afterward, my charge nurse took me aside and verbally reprimanded me for breaking confidentiality. Because my breach was innocent, she told me, she'd let it go that once; I was never to vent my feelings to anyone outside our unit again.

I've since wondered what would have happened if another tech had been assigned to the woman we'd restrained that night, or if the assigned tech had simply let her storm to her room. The incident had nothing to do with therapy; it was a power struggle over the line between staff and patients, which was clearly drawn from the moment we walked through the doors with keys denied to the patients. Looking back on that night, years later, I wonder what could have prompted us to show more compassion than power. What personal story might we have known about the woman's life that would have helped us to lead her toward the cathartic tears, bypassing the seclusion and restraints? At the time, I was lost with a different question: why had my charge nurse forbidden me to discuss my *feelings* with those outside of work? Were they too closely entangled with the events and patients of the unit? Was it wrong to describe incidents, even without names, because others could potentially infer who I was talking about? And what if I didn't feel comfortable discussing my feelings with my coworkers—people I barely knew?

The whole ordeal, from hotdog binge to embarrassing reprimand, stayed with me throughout nursing school and into my years as a novice nurse. I was careful to share little about those whom I cared for, partly because I was overly conscious of my duty to keep quiet, partly because it was never clear to me what could be acceptably shared outside of work. Names were out, obviously, but what about conversations? I felt fairly certain that I could talk about medical conditions ("the bowel obstruction in room 234") and medical tasks ("I had trouble getting a Foley catheter in one woman tonight"), but diagnoses and assigned chores weren't always what I wanted to talk about. There was the other stuff about my job—the stories that patients shared with me, the dynamics I witnessed between family members. So many of my patients shared their physical and emotional vulnerabilities with me not so much by choice as by circumstance. What did I do with that?

Fortunately, I stumbled upon a job in a small endoscopy unit—just a room, really, that was crammed between some offices and the operating room suites. There, in that small space, in the closed-door quiet, spontaneous admissions would emerge from strangers. My patients would share their fears, I would reassure them and make them laugh or smile, and the conversation would turn to something private, personal, and desperately heartbreaking: their cancer, a child's death, their boyfriend troubles. I loved to listen. At the end of the day, as my colleagues and I cleaned or caught up on charting, I'd retell my patients' stories to the other two nurses. I wanted to share their narratives, to extend the touch of their beliefs or experiences out to an ever-expanding spiral that says: *This is what we can learn from each other.*

It was also a way to undo the day. By remembering the funny and sad things someone had said, by mixing them in with the complicated lung brushings, the hassle of subtraction errors on the narcotic count, and the biting comments from "that nurse on Three North," I washed the day's events from my thoughts like I used soap to slide bacteria from my hands. I could share these stories so long as I shared them only with my colleagues. We were in it together. It made sense to vent to each other, to unburden ourselves, and then to go home clean.

I unloaded not only the stories I heard, but also the events I witnessed. Like the time a teenager claimed to have sat on a wide piece of plastic, which we then spent an hour extracting from his rectum. A surgeon with extra tools came to help, while I pleaded with the doctors to consider further treatment for pain. "One more of Versed, twenty-five more of fentanyl?"

The gastroenterologist and the surgeon refused to completely knock the kid out in the emergency room, and I looked into his flat eyes and tight lips that betrayed his embarrassment. "I'm all right," he kept insisting when I asked, but I wanted to push enough drugs for both of us to forget that moment, to forget his quest for pleasure that had twisted into a pain we thought would need surgical removal. Retelling moments like these helps me to let them go.

When I later transferred to another department, I developed a similar feeling of camaraderie with my new coworkers; more stories were exchanged. I began visualizing my patients as bodies of literature—good books waiting to be read, passed on, and talked about with others. No one else could help me to unburden myself of my workday, and I needed this outlet. Without it, the stories would surely stack up on each other, build up inside of me, echo in flashes, and fray like heat lightning in my dry mind. They would haunt me as amplified memories. A patient's experience was my experience as well; we entered into it together, but the patient owned it. I didn't.

When HIPAA's privacy rules went into effect in April of 2003, terms like *individually identifiable* and *protected health information* (PHI) were introduced as a means to establish uniform standards for the acquisition, use, and exchange of *health information data,* which could be shared only on a need-to-know basis. No one, unless that person were directly involved with either care or payment, was to know anything about anyone. These new regulations came coupled with a universal fear that the US Department of Health and Human Services would jail or fine us for—for what? For casually sharing with a coworker some lab result, some tidbit of information she didn't need to know because she wasn't directly caring for the patient?

So much for sharing stories. So much for sharing anything with anybody. *Individually identifiable* included any data that could potentially point to a specific person: demographics, symptoms, diagnosis, or treatments. The nurse working next to me was not supposed to know whom I was taking care of or why unless the patient's care required the nurse to know. My coworkers and I considered this point to be particularly crazy. While the law acted as the noble protector of the patient, it ignored the support network that nurses had built together, as well as the individual uplift a communal experience engenders. When something unpleasant happens, nurses turn to each other for validation and the knowledge that we all have bad days. It also ignored the shared burden of telling a story. I remembered my days in endoscopy, where I could recount the stories I'd heard and the moments I'd worked through and let them slide off me before I went home. HIPAA may have been good for patients, but it pulled the sink away from me, and I was left with no place to wash my hands.

Inservices were created to educate us on the new law: Get Hip to HIPAA. I began to think of it as a child on my hip, one that was too unwieldy to handle and hold. I *had* understood the importance of upholding a patient's legal right to privacy, how it established rapport and preserved trust. In our town of fifty thousand, I took care of a lot of familiar community members, which meant that even my husband, a social worker who also understood the rules, sometimes found himself in awkward positions. Arriving home on one occasion, he told me, "I saw John and Jackie at the farmers' market."

"How are they doing?" I said.

"They had their baby. They acted like I already knew because you did."

"Oh. I wasn't her nurse. I never asked if I could tell you."

"I wasn't sure if I'd get you in trouble if I pretended you had told me, or if I should risk hurting their feelings by telling them you hadn't."

"What'd you say?"

"I told them I had to leave."

One of the most awkward times for us both was when his professor came in for a colonoscopy. I was the sedation nurse. I referred to his girlfriend as his daughter (she was many years younger than he), and my husband felt he'd been placed in an uncomfortable position when his professor later complained to him about it. For me, the discomfort came later, when my husband and I attended a party at their house. I acted as if it were the first time I'd met the man, but he soon asked me about the polyps I'd helped remove from his colon, and before long everyone at the party knew I'd been his nurse. For a patient, this may mean little. Patients can say whatever they want about their experiences with me, but I'm not allowed to share the experiences I've had with them.

It's like waking up to eat breakfast with all the family members of a one-night stand. It means I've shared something intimate with a stranger I'd planned never to see again. But then I hear, "She was my nurse," and I feel pressured to act in a certain way, as if we're still in a setting with certain rules. People I know from a public context strip from their street clothes, don the homogenized identity parceled out with the ubiquitous gowns, slip into bed sheets, and trust me implicitly. I observe them in postures they hide from their closest friends. I learn facts I sometimes wish I hadn't and consequently know these people differently when we meet again in public.

Of course, HIPAA's job isn't to protect me. It is to protect patients, and I have seen the ugly other side where healthcare workers abused their positions. In one hospital where I worked as a nurse, the electronic charting system made most of the information about patients in one area of the hospital available to staff in another, unrelated one. Some of my peers tracked how busy the emergency department was, discovering who was admitted and why. How many drunks? What was the trauma? One of my coworkers, a unit secretary, preferred pediatrics over emergency medicine; she'd look up what the kids were in for, then decide which child had the worst parents. Some nurses liked to see how many patients had abortions before they decided to keep a child, an informal survey with character discussions following each find. When a well-known hospital employee stroked, everyone in the hospital knew about it. Any interested person could find out what medications he was receiving and track his progress throughout his hospital stay.

Administrators frowned upon these practices. But patients are not described in ink and pressed inside folders like they once were; their medical records are no longer stored safely in one room or behind one gatekeeper. Instead, they switch through wires, spreading like gossip, where the patient's privacy can be disclosed to or discovered by many people who don't need the information but want it. Before HIPAA, our computer systems didn't have reliable ways to control access. Peeping was relatively easy and safe. HIPAA unplugged this open-information effect of electronic documentation and file storage.

The fact remains that patients are vulnerable, and healthcare workers do have access to privileged information. But outside of this (and to return to the context of storytelling), at what point is individually identifiable health information, like a breast cancer diagnosis, also a universally identifiable experience? The physical and mental history of one individual may be very similar to the physical and mental histories of a thousand other people. Sharing one person's story is a way of connecting to another's.

There was another woman whom I helped. She had a slow leak from a blood vessel that was nicked during surgery. Before anyone knew about the vessel, her nurse had paged the doctor multiple times about the patient's abdominal pain and ashy color. She begged the nurses, "Please, help me," through pale lips that were drying like fish scales in the sun. The doctor was with his family at the county fair. He strolled onto the unit, sunburned and smiling, evaluated the patient, and ordered a CT scan; it had been hours since he'd admitted her by phone. By the time the abdominal leak was identified, the surgeon didn't want to open her up—the release of the pressure on the defect could cause the small hole to tear open, allowing her blood to leak out faster than the hole could be identified and sewn shut. The surgeon explained this to her, detailed her probable death in the operating room, and then smiled and said, "Here's the option that I like."

He explained how excited he was by the idea: at a certain point, there wouldn't be any room in the abdominal cavity for more blood, which might eventually create enough pressure to close the hole for him. The other nurses and I raised our eyebrows at each other. At the nurses' station, we whispered our disbelief. The patient's heart was pumping blood to the wrong place and slowly killing her; her breath was rasping, her belly was rigid from the blood pressing her organs tight, and we were going to wait and see if she could make it, wait and see if her own blood would tamponade the slow leak and stop it.

Her blood pressure dropped almost moments after he had told her that it probably would. When it kept dropping—80 over 50, 70 over 40, 60 over 30—it became clear that the surgeon's avoidance of surgery hadn't worked, and we ran her to the emergency department ("Faster, faster!" the surgeon yelled at us, "she's going to die in the hall!"), where they treated her like a fresh trauma. They started new lines using the largest bore tubes possible, as big as would fit in her vessels, and expanded her circulatory volume, enabling her heart to continue pumping red blood cells throughout her body. The lab arrived with a box of blood that hadn't been crossed to match her blood type, increasing her risk of suffering a mortal reaction.

"Please, don't leave me," she said to those whose hands she could grasp, feeling the elusive and tricky slipping away of her life. I stayed with her in the trauma room until she was ready to let go of our hands and place her trust in the oncoming rush, the volume of blood from other people. I left her surrounded by a new group of caretakers who filled her body with what could save her more than our holding hands. She never had the surgery. She spent days in critical care and was eventually discharged from the hospital. But she never left me, and she never left the others. We found ourselves turning back to her in conversations that took place months and years later, still upset by the experience. Her experience was ours too. But she owns it like a copyright. And what do we, the nurses, own? The universal experience: the near-death experience. This is the balance I have found for myself with HIPAA.

There was another woman who needed a box of blood. Her baby had died inside of her, and the doctor on call didn't want to pull them apart. He kept her waiting until morning so he could stay in bed and catch some extra sleep. The nurses called him repeatedly, but he refused to see the patient before he arrived for morning rounds. By then she needed twenty-eight units of packed red blood cells, plus fresh, frozen plasma. The usual transfusion is two units. At one unit of whole blood per donation, that's twenty-eight people who ate cookies and gave two cups. With four cups in a quart and approximately five quarts in the average body, it was enough donated blood to provide nearly three people with their total blood volume.

Blood is thicker than water due to its millions of suspended cells. Too thick, it clots. When clotting factors (proteins that form blood clots) fail, blood runs too thin. The woman who lost her baby had blood like that—it was loose because of a condition known as disseminated intravascular coagulopathy (DIC). The body can endure a certain amount of rapid blood loss by slowing things down with clotting factors. It's like adding mesh or cheesecloth to the spout of a funneled container or like mixing particles into the liquid being poured. The more particles, the slower the flow. In a hemorrhage, however, too many clotting factors are sent out and used up. This signals a chemical warning that the blood is forming too many clots; thinning factors (clot busters) are released, which in turn causes instability in the whole hemodynamic system. The balance gets lost. The patient's blood pressure drops dangerously low, the heart beats too fast, and oxygen is not moving into tissues as the body goes into shock. When water boils, the water will boil itself out of the pot if the heat isn't turned down. That's DIC. That's what happened to the dead boy's mother while the physician took extra time to sleep.

He was a perfect boy, full term, even if he was blue. We wrapped him in blankets and hid him in a bassinet behind the nurse's station until the staff who wanted to see him—how beautiful he would have been—could do so before we enclosed him in the baby refrigerator. I think back on that moment as the boy's first funeral. The nurses came and paid their respects. We shared our anger at the physician and the experience by expressing our grief for the child.

I arrived home two hours later than usual. My husband was angry. We had a baby of our own at that time, and he had expected me home with fresh milk. "Why didn't you call?" he asked.

All I could say was that there had been a patient who almost died. "They needed help. I needed to stay. I'm sorry," I said.

When I went back to work that night, the tech who had assisted the obstetricians during the C-section told me that the patient's blood had never clotted. Outside the body, blood thickens and dries. Two hours after the trauma, the tech had returned to the room to clean and restock when she saw the never-dumped bowl of blood and feared how hard it would be to scour. "Two hours of sitting, and I thought it was going to be oozed gel," she said. "But it poured right out as if it had never sat there."

The things I had read about in textbooks—hypofibrinogenemia, prolonged prothrombin time, disseminated intravascular coagulopathy, abruptio placentae, dead fetus syndrome—had become real. How could I *not* need to talk about them with someone? According to the law, that burden on my hip, I'm in violation if I discuss someone's care with anyone who doesn't need to know. No one should have seen the dead baby unless the viewing was necessary in order to provide adequate care. HIPAA, however, does not consider a nurse's need to process feelings of fear, grief, helplessness, or anger—emotions that will prevent us from sleeping when we go home. Nurses need to feel that they can talk to each other and their loved ones about upsetting experiences without the threat of being penalized. When a law like HIPAA is passed—one that grants patients the power to limit the disclosure of their information—the message, to me, is that I can't be trusted with their stories, that patients need boundaries and protections from me and what I know. The law tells me I can be dangerous to the patient, but I already know this. It was drilled into me in nursing school.

Again, I think back to the space I had in endoscopy, where the days' events were shared and let go. That small room where patients felt enough security to open up had been a storage closet before it was cleaned out and used for procedures. It makes me wonder what other spaces could be cleared for nurses and patients. Without this sharing, like the blood that didn't clot, these barriers of law, power, and need will never resolve.

So much exists between a patient and a care provider: disease, viruses, pain, surgery, rooms, and gloves. Patient loads, acuity statuses, call lights, coworkers, and bosses. And so much doesn't. There is little between us: white sheets, finger pads, a stethoscope membrane, a port into the bloodstream. I read their bodies like stories, touching their skin and smoothing out the ripples between what I overhear and what they choose to confide. I've decided that the story I know is stitched along with each suture, pinned beneath each staple, and glued shut under the liquid plastic of a collodion-sealed incision:

each person is her own body of literature that waits to be spoken. The words can remain with the patients, flaking off in dead skin cells left behind for only the mites to mouth, or they can be given their own space to be shared.

Knowing someone's story helps to make the patient more real, and it makes the job more personal. What else didn't we know about the naked, restrained woman? What else about her would have made us more compassionate? We surely wouldn't have done that to our daughters, our mothers, or our aunts. Why? Because of the mutual, shared stories we have with these people. It's what cements us together. The shared narratives of others' lives incorporate and become stories about us. I feel myself to be a part of a stranger's story, when it is shared with me, and passing it on feels like my sharing of a parable we've all heard—we know the plot, even the climax and the ending. Only the names have changed, or the costumes, or the settings, but the story is the same and is this: we are all vulnerable; we are all a little bit crazy; we are all funny, entertaining, delicate, bold, horrible, and fantastic. We are all, in our unique and individual ways, as equally and universally fucked up as the next person. Every one of us. There's comfort in knowing this.

PAMELA BAKER *received her MFA in creative writing from the University of Central Florida in Orlando, where she currently works as a nurse. Her nonfiction has been published in* The Journal, Bayou Magazine, *and* Cream City Review.

APPROACHING DEATH

Kimberly A. Condon

A nurse working in a fast-paced emergency room develops a simple strategy for coping with the tragedies and traumas she sees everyday: "Build walls and stay busy." She discovers, however, that the rapid pace of nursing can sometimes prevent necessary reflection.

A child is dead.

There is a terrifying, soul-piercing scream that a mother makes when she loses a child. This scream is so universal that everyone, in every corner of the emergency department, knows what has just happened when they hear it.

On a sunny summer morning, a young mother of a three-year-old watched, stunned by ultimate dread, as her little boy ran out into the normally quiet street. On that day, however, the driver of a rainbow-painted Volkswagen bus careened through the neighborhood; twenty minutes later the mother stood in our trauma room, looking as if she might collapse. She told us, through tears and broken English, how she had heard the screech of tires, the crumpling thud. She ran into the street, knelt down to her son, and gathered the little boy into her arms.

It may have been clear to the paramedics, when they arrived, that this child had no life left in him, yet they knew to move with the kind of energy that infuses hope into impossible situations. They did everything in their power—oxygen, monitors, IVs—an all-out resuscitative effort. It is hard to imagine anything worse for a parent than to watch an aggressive attempt at her child's resuscitation. Except, I suppose, to see no effort at all.

The little, broken body was transported to our emergency room, and we put on a similar show—a collective swoop of doctors and nurses and technicians. We focused the exam lights on him and looked, listened, strained to detect some tiny morsel of life with which to run; it's not just for the benefit of the parents that we go all out, even when mottling has set in. We, too, need this cathartic effort in order to begin to grieve. Seeing a child die is never easy.

Years ago, it was customary to keep families out of the room when a crisis was in progress. But nowadays we know that one last look, one more moment of hope can be vitally important to the process of saying good-bye. The mother, looking stricken and white, stood by the door and held onto the arm of a nurse. When the initial moments had passed, the chaotic energy in the room suddenly changed. The doctor lowered his voice and called the time.

And so, the scream.

I left the room to find the father in the waiting room down the hall. I paused at the door before entering, wanting to wait as long as possible before destroying his world. He took one look at my face and fell to his knees, his forehead slapping onto the scuffed white floor. I waited while he groaned to his feet, then led him to his wife and dead child. So the parents could sit with the little boy, the team had tried to clean him up and had pulled the tube from his nose. I motioned the father into the room and left them alone to say their good-byes. I had to rush to the next emergency.

That was the moment when my edges began to wither, and I felt a hardness creeping in. Was it really possible that my response to the intense anguish of two broken parents was to push them into a room and run off to finish my job? When had I become so callous? I remembered myself as a new nurse—one who made it a point to touch every patient, even when she wasn't examining them; who had a gift for sensing what a psychotic patient needed in order to de-escalate; who was known as the one to call when a battered woman needed to feel safe enough to talk—but this memory was distant and faded.

I was overly sensitive, even as a child, to the suffering of others. When I watched Westerns, I would get teary when the cowboys yanked at the mouths of their horses. "Think about how lucky those horses are," my father had said, trying to console me, "They get to run all day." I became so upset when I read *Black Beauty* that I hid in my room and cried for hours. I know the story has a happy ending only from secondhand accounts, as I've never been able to bring myself to finish it. In the fourth grade, I jokingly pulled the chair out from behind a shy and quiet classmate, the way I had seen it done on the Three Stooges. The boy fell and hurt his back, and I was so distraught over his tears that I never spoke to him again. While working in a bookstore, years later, I happened to glance through the pages of an autobiography written by a man who had been viciously abused as a child. I went home sick that day because I simply couldn't function with those pictures in my head.

How does someone with these pathological, debilitating reactions to distress function in a world of endless pain and struggle? Easy. Build walls and stay busy.

I had been involved in emergency medicine for fourteen years—first as an emergency medical technician, then as a paramedic, and finally as a nurse. The crackling energy and hot, white lights of the ER seemed like a perfect fit for my frenetic nature. I'd always had enormous reserves of energy; reading was the only thing that ever slowed my racing thoughts, and my mother would hand me a book the way another might hand her child a lollipop. So, there I was, a center-stage participant in a vital dance, and the result was a matter of life and death. I felt completely at ease. When I speed-walked down the halls, I often heard the joke, "Where's the fire?" There were never charts waiting on the desk when I was working, and my inability to sit still, or even to slow down, lessened the workload for everyone as I zipped through the incidentals, the standard protocols, the well-worn paths of action. Everyone around me thought I was doing a great job.

But nonstop motion is not always as productive as it seems—the best emergency workers, in fact, move slowly, carefully. I eventually realized I was missing something. I felt like I was floating through someone else's life, as if I wasn't actually feeling compassion. I felt like a fraud.

I went to nursing school partly because I liked being the one whom people looked to and leaned on in times of crisis. Like many people I met in emergency medicine, I had the proverbial need to be needed. I took pride in caring for my patients, but my urgency to be in the next moment prevented me from really seeing them. My coworkers liked to work with me, of course, and my employers thought I was excelling. But what about the patients? I didn't know how to find my buried compassion, nor did I know what to do next. But I knew the time had come to move on.

The ability to change specialties is one of the best aspects of nursing. I assumed, because I had seen so much, because my critical-care skills were the envy of some physicians, and because I knew exactly how to react in the direst of situations, that I was qualified to do anything. I had seen things most people would never see, having been at the center of a pounding, bloody battle where we won as often as we lost. I needed something completely different. Of course, any other type of nursing would be, if not a step down, at least less challenging. I walked around a job fair, aimless and uncertain, until I found myself standing in front of a hospice booth.

I had been, in my childhood, a distant witness to several deaths. When my great-grandfather died, I watched my mom cry and was sad he would never finish teaching me to play pinochle. I was heartbroken for my friend when her mother died, and I cried and cried when a car hit my golden retriever. But I was never afraid. This is not to say that I was evolved or anything. When I was thirteen years old and square in the middle of that most awkward, terrifying slice of adolescence, I actually looked forward to death. Perhaps it was a brief, pathological, adolescence-induced depression that made me wish for it. As I matured, however, the feeling that death was a lovely way out stayed with me. Nothing could ever get me really down, or be too serious, because I would eventually die. It may sound like a strange consolation, but I had become quite comfortable with my old friend, Death.

Maybe hospice would be the fit I was searching for. During my first month of the new job, I agreed to work the weekend on-call shift. Two twelve-hour days of nonstop calls took me from one end of the spectrum to the other: reinsert a urinary catheter, teach a family what CPR really entails, hold a child's hand as his mother takes her final breaths. I constantly switched gears, depending on where a particular patient or family happened to fall on the timeline of life and death. Caring for the dying, as well as their families, I hardly noticed that I had somehow chosen the one shift in hospice that fit my old profile.

Over one weekend, I ordered antibiotics for a ninety-eight-year-old woman who lived alone and refused help with anything, comforted a woman who had to place her elderly husband in a nursing home against his will, and started an IV on a young woman who insisted she was not ready to die, though every system in her body was decaying from cancer. I spent two hours talking a wildly delirious patient into allowing his wife to give him his meds; I ran back to the office for supplies, twice; and I spent several hours with family members as they waited for the mortuary to pick up their matriarch.

It was five o'clock on a crisp, chilly Sunday evening when my pager beeped again: "Six-week-old patient in crisis."

Six weeks?

A tiny flaw in the genetic makeup of a developing human can result in a life just incomplete enough—after nine months of gestating, sixteen hours of birthing, and a few hours of bonding—to be afflicted with multiple congenital anomalies. "Take him home," the doctors said, "and hospice will help you keep him comfortable. We are probably talking about weeks."

The baby would suffer from longer and longer periods of status epilepticus, and drugs would become less and less effective. His tiny frame would flail in violent, disorganized muscle contractions ten, fifteen, twenty times a day. The hospice team—a nurse, a social worker, a chaplain, and a CNA—visited the parents every day to comfort them, to teach them to care for him, and to support their grieving process. The family had gotten to know this team, but I was the nurse on call that day.

Thirty minutes after I got the page, I drove up a bumpy dirt road to a little green house on the side of a mountain. The neighborhood was quiet, private, and filled with golden aspens changing colors for the season. The door opened before I knocked. The father's eyes were teary, and his parchment skin looked drained and hollow. He led me silently through a hallway, one entire wall of which was covered with books—perhaps the ones they had hoped their son would read. The mother was sitting in a rocking chair, holding her seizing infant. "It hasn't stopped for twelve minutes."

All I could do for him, for them, was be calm and present as this tiny creature worked his way toward the end we all come to. My heart broke for them, but I stood by and fought the urge to rush in. I couldn't intrude on this precious process. I waited with them, moving only to help with positioning or to offer gentle suggestions. In the air, I felt his tiny presence slip away, slowly and peacefully. He stopped moving, his breathing slowed until it was imperceptible, and for a moment his complete stillness made me hold my own breath. I reached for the pediatric stethoscope around my neck, warming it in my hand so as not to startle him. As I pressed it against his chest, his mother said, "His name is Christopher."

"Hi, Christopher," I whispered as I listened.

I didn't need to say the words. I knew from her expression that she knew. A slow, fat tear dripped down her face, and I backed away, just far enough out of the picture, in my attempt not to invade this moment of good-bye between the three of them. There was nothing for me to do but be still. I crept back, found a chair, and sat to wait.

And then I began to sob.

I felt myself losing control, choking and sobbing as if he were my child, my loss. I didn't even have children. I tried not to make noise, tried not to trespass on their moment. I was so ashamed! I was supposed to be their support, their rock. I moved to quietly slip out of the room, but I felt the husband's hand on my shoulder. His eyes were wet and kind. He handed me a tissue.

I couldn't believe what a failure I was.

I got it together, finally, and helped them decide what to do. I called the physician, the coroner, and the mortuary. At the mother's request, I got permission from the mortuary for the couple to drive the tiny body themselves. I helped them into the car by holding the baby, who now had a little blue cap on his head, while his mother settled herself in the passenger's seat. I placed Christopher on her lap, hoping they wouldn't get pulled over and have to explain why their baby was not in a car seat.

I was watching them ease down the driveway when the car suddenly stopped. The mother gently handed her little bundle over to her husband and got out of the car. Before I could react, she'd wrapped her arms around me. I was so stunned by the gentle, intimate comfort she offered that I barely moved. She finally let me go, looked at me, and then got back into the car. They drove off. As I watched them go, I wondered if maybe I hadn't failed. I hadn't swallowed my grief. I hadn't patronized them or tried to explain "the process." I had been absolutely present with them in that agonizing, priceless moment. It was the best I could do.

KIMBERLY A. CONDON *graduated from the University of Wisconsin–Madison and has spent twenty years in the field of medicine, both as a nurse and as a paramedic. She writes in North Carolina, where she lives with her partner on a horse farm.*

THE NURSES WHISPERED

Patricia A. Nugent

Our parents' deaths can confront us with some of the most difficult decisions we'll ever make. Here, a daughter pays tribute to the nurses who steadfastly offered their compassion, guidance, and support during the final eighteen months of her parents' lives.

It was the doctor who told us, in a neutral and matter-of-fact tone, that it was time to refer my father to hospice. It was he who sat down with us in the cold, sterile hospital environment to lay it on the line, to tell us there was no hope. "We'll do what we have to do," my mother replied stoically, looking simultaneously sad and radiant. Just a few weeks before, they had gone for a walk, and he had fallen and broken his hip. Anesthesia and hip replacement surgery had left him weakened and unable to swallow correctly.

The doctors tried to convince my mother to allow a feeding tube. She called me from the Florida hospital. "They want to put a feeding tube in your father. I said no, but they say they must." She was more unglued than I'd ever heard her and desperately looking for direction from me—a rare occurrence. "Your father won't tolerate a feeding tube," she continued. "He'll tear it out. He'd rather die than live like that. I can't let them do this to him. They keep sending different doctors in to try to convince me. But one nurse whispered to me that I was right, that she wouldn't do it either. And I won't."

The nurse who'd had the courage to whisper in my mother's ear that day, when both my sister and I were living out of state, made all the difference.

Thanks to her informal counsel, my mother stuck to her guns and insisted that my father not receive a feeding tube. Instead, he received speech therapy to improve his swallowing; he eventually graduated out of hospice, living another eighteen months. He would live long enough to witness the passing of his best healthcare advocate, his wife.

A few months after that phone conversation with my mother, it was a doctor who told us, in bold declarative statements, that my mother had brain cancer. "I have the biopsy results. I'll meet you in the conference room to discuss them," the neurosurgeon said. I hung up the phone in the nurses' station, numb but fully aware of the implication. A face-to-face meeting with a busy neurosurgeon signaled a negative outcome. I could see the conference room from where I stood but didn't know if my legs could carry me there. The nurses hugged me, whispering in my ear that it would be OK. The doctor arrived and took a seat; I remained standing. "Not only is it malignant," he said, "but it is also aggressive. Radiation will help." I barely heard him. I realized that I was alone in the room only when a nurse came to get me sometime later. She stayed while I sobbed over the news I'd been given, offering words of encouragement and hope.

My mother endured the radiation, though she said it was squeezing all her brains out, and she endured what she called the "seismic pounding" of repeated MRIs. She withstood these procedures because the doctor said they would help. Her paralysis grew worse by the day, and the nurses struggled to turn and move her, exerting much physical energy to keep her comfortable. The nurses also worked to keep her spirits high during this time.

"It's a lousy diagnosis with a lousy prognosis," another doctor said after the thirty-two radiation treatments were completed. "No more interventions are called for." It was the nurses who whispered, "We will do everything we can to make her comfortable." And they did. Yet, due to staffing shortages, I frequently ended up waiting and watching in the hallway as the overworked nurses passed me by. I would try to get their attention, but I also realized that I couldn't be too bold or demanding; there were many family members standing in the hallway, and we were all dependent on those nurses who cared for our loved ones. Doctors making their rounds walked by, but few of us had the courage to stop them. But the nurses kept a steady pace, often working extended shifts with large and severe caseloads. They looked exhausted but did everything they could to accommodate requests. So many requests.

They toileted, washed, dressed, fed, kissed, and loved my mother. Most important, they accepted the person she had become as a result of her illness—it was the kindest of gestures. They didn't reflect back to her any pain, disappointment, or frustration with her decline like her family did, those who knew how capable she had once been. Instead, they emanated total acceptance and support. They modeled a mindset, teaching me both to accept my mother as she was and to cease wishing for the return of my "real" mom.

My mother clung tightly to the hospice nurse's hand during their first visit to her nursing home room. She was a very private person, and I had never dreamed she'd be willing to confide in a stranger. Yet she told the nurse of the traumatic radiation treatments, describing them in detail. And I heard her whisper, when she thought I was out of earshot, "I need more support. I need more *outside* support. Do you know what I mean?" I heard the nurse whisper that she would be there for my mother, that she would be the support my mother needed. Despite my daily presence at her bedside, she needed more comfort than I could provide. She needed to speak openly about her fears and feelings without the worry of upsetting her family. Try as I might, I was not enough. That hospice nurse would serve as my mother's true confidante for the rest of her life.

When you spend so much time in elder care facilities, you get to know the other residents and patients; they become part of your extended family, and I had the privilege to observe the nurses' relationships with them. One day, two nurses went to see my mother's ninety-year-old roommate together, knowing that reinforcement would be needed. True to form, she was ready for them. They gently tried to talk her into a tuberculosis test, a hearing aid, a flu shot—she declined them all, with attitude. Then they asked more significant questions. "You haven't been eating very much, Peggy. Are you depressed? Have you given up?"

"My dear nurses, it is simply that I am already too old," Peggy responded. "May I take a nap now?" They whispered soothing words of understanding and respectfully left. I could tell that while they'd done what they'd had to do, they had also supported Peggy's decision to decline intervention.

Despite my mother's terminal condition, she was scheduled for another MRI, a procedure she had grown to strongly dislike. I wasn't sure whether to proceed or not. What if additional information could be gleaned that might suggest a different course of treatment? What if a miracle had occurred? I was stymied, unable to say "yes" or "no." A nurse came and sat with me. So neither my mother nor the doctors would hear, she whispered that she didn't support the scan, which would require my mother to be transported by ambulance to the radiation center; it would put her through unnecessary trauma while changing nothing. I felt at peace and told my mother that she wouldn't be subjected to any more tests or treatment. She, too, felt at peace. The nurse had made an agonizing decision easier.

When her time came, there were no monitors or beeping gadgets to tell us that her life was leaving—just real people who took her pulse, listened to her heart, looked at her. Real people who assessed the best interests of a real person who was dying. The nurses whispered to me the indicators that death was near; when they examined her, they told me what they were looking for. I didn't know whether to hope for the presence or absence of these indicators. I passively watched the nurses, scared to hear their reports. The oxygen machine hummed loudly in the room, reminding us that her condition was worsening. But I didn't need a machine to tell me she was leaving. The nurses closely monitored us both. They were the first ones on the scene when I awoke on the cot next to my mother's bed that morning and realized she was gone. They were the first to offer condolences.

•   •   •

My parents had been placed in different facilities based on room availability and their specific medical needs. While my mother was alive, I spent my days with her and then rushed off to visit my father by night. His little room was a stop on the way home. Too often, he was already sleeping when I snuck in through the employee entrance; the nurses had whispered to me this secret way of getting in after visiting hours. They knew it was better for my father to get a good-night kiss from a loved one than to toss and turn in a fist-clenched sleep. The night was a little less dark thanks to the nurses who looked the other way, permitting me to crawl into bed and comfort the lonely man. They never asked me to leave—they even slipped me cookies.

Yet the stress of caregiving for two parents was sometimes too much. One day, my father and I were in his room, screaming at each other. *Screaming.* He wanted to get out of there, to go home. He asked why his wife never came to see him; he asked if there was "someone else." I was at my wit's end, torn between two desperate parents whose lives had come unraveled so suddenly. "Mom has a brain tumor, Dad!" I screamed back at him. "A brain tumor! She's dying, OK? Can't you think about someone else for a change?" I instantly regretted having told him in that way; it had just slipped out. For months I had tried to shield him from the grim reality of his wife's impending death. My deception weighed heavily on me, but my disclosure didn't seem to have any impact on him now.

The head nurse suddenly appeared and began to calm us down, gently whispering words of comfort to my father. She suggested that I leave, saying she'd take care of him. I quickly gathered my stuff and ran down the hall, crying. I heard him yelling after me with his booming voice, "Get me out of here! Patty? Get me out of here!" Between his outbursts, I could hear the nurse as she continued to whisper gentle, calming words. "Why can't I relate to him like that?" I thought. "She's better with my own father than I am!" The nurses clearly provided more than just medical procedures.

A few days later, a woman with jet-black hair walked into the little room where I was sitting with my dad. She told us to watch out for athlete's foot in the shower and not to leave valuables lying around. She was animated and spoke with great authority, so I assumed she was a new employee. We told her we'd be careful; she reminded us once more before leaving. And then again. I followed her out and was told by an aide that her name was Mary, that she was once a nurse on that floor, and that she was now a patient. Many times afterward, I sat and chatted with Mary about the work she'd done several decades ago— something she could remember much better than more recent events. "It was hard work," she said. "My back hurt. But I enjoyed helping people who needed me." She struggled to accept that she was now the one in need.

Erin was a young, red-haired nurse with a personality that wonderfully counterbalanced my father's grumpiness. She brightened the dark nights by always greeting me with a smile, no matter how exhausted she was from her demanding work. She told me I was a good daughter, something I desperately needed to hear. "In fact," she said, "you're one of the best." Erin cheered up my dad when he was hurting and validated my concerns about his medication when the doctor was dismissive or unreachable. She took the time to look in my dad's chart to answer my questions. She made us feel as if we were in good hands, regardless of how busy she was. She helped to keep my dad alive through tough times and consoled me when it was time for him to take his leave.

One morning, ten months after being told that his wife of sixty-three years was dead, my father refused food and drink, ripped off his oxygen mask, and spit out the antibiotic they tried to give him. He belligerently told the nurses, "No more" and "Get away" and "That's enough." I told him he would get better if he took the pills. "I don't care," he responded.

"Do you want to go to the hospital?" I asked repeatedly. He declined emphatically every time. My father's nurse told me that the doctor was refusing to prescribe any more morphine and might have to send my father to the hospital for antibiotics to treat pneumonia and, possibly, for tube feeding, as he was again having difficulty swallowing. I panicked, remembering my mother's phone call from the Florida hospital eighteen months earlier. I could not allow him to have a feeding tube now. The nurses whispered to me that rather than attempting heroic interventions, it would be more peaceful for him to die in his own room with those who had cared for him for more than a year. They gave me the strength and courage to advocate that this ninety-year-old man with dementia not be whisked off to a strange environment. Although I lost that battle, the nurses were by my side all the while, whispering words of encouragement as I challenged the doctors and the medical establishment. I'll never forget their sad faces as they watched my father being put into an ambulance; he weakly waved to them. He died three days later.

Nurses were there every step of the way during my parents' eighteen-month journey from life to death. They were there for both my parents and for me. They had different styles, different faces, different specialties, but one trait was the same: they provided quiet, behind-the-scenes support and guidance to a family in trouble. They were assertive when the situation demanded it. When we didn't know what to do or where to turn, they were brave enough to give us counsel based on humanistic concern and personal experience. Counsel drawn not exclusively from volumes of medical journals and training but from their intimate experiences with families. They were not afraid of personal or professional liability when offering an opinion, but they whispered to avoid offending those with whom they disagreed. (It is well-known that many doctors do not like to be challenged.) During these desperate times in our lives, their whisperings seemed like the messages of angels. Such whisperings gave us the grace to keep going and the knowledge we needed to make informed decisions under duress. I will forever hold their service in gratitude, and I write this in their honor.

Patricia A. Nugent *is the author of* They Live On: Saying Goodbye to Mom and Dad, *a compilation of vignettes portraying the stages of caring for and saying good-bye to a loved one. She has been published in national professional journals and has received awards for her creative nonfiction essays, including one bestowed by Susan Sontag. She has served as a teacher, administrator, adjunct professor, and consultant.*

BECOMING

Lori Mulvihill

"Nurses have a longstanding tradition of eating their young," reflects a veteran Ob-gyn nurse, remembering the inexperienced student she once was, as well as the tough love that made her a better nurse.

The hospital feels larger than life. Oppressive. Or maybe it's my anxiety that's large and oppressive. The stiff, white fabric of my new uniform has been washed but never worn. It crinkles when I walk. The stethoscope around my neck is only a prop. I don't know much about using it. STUDENT, my name badge announces. It might as well say IMPOSTER. I feel like I'm at my elementary school's Halloween parade except for the lack of candy and joviality. A party atmosphere this is not.

I peer tentatively into the dimly lit room, ready to play my part, or rather, to *find* my part. Her slight frame makes the hospital bed look huge. Her wide, deep brown eyes—not vacant, exactly, but not totally present either—make her bruised face look small. Her skin is mottled with bruises, her gray hair unkempt. Her inner-city Detroit home was broken into, and she was beaten so badly by the intruders that she had cardiac contusions; her heart was bruised. Not broken, but bruised. My heart feels a bit bruised, too. Our anxious eyes meet. She allows me to help her to the bathroom, brush her hair, and change her linens. It's the extent of my patient care knowledge. It feels awkward to touch a person this way: intimate, yet detached.

No small part of me wants to run screaming from the building. I can't do this. What am I thinking, getting this close to the suffering of others? I can't fix it. What do they want from me? I'm just a naïve young mother from a college town in Colorado. My baby is in day care, and being away from her feels like missing a limb. Biochemistry, organic chemistry, and microbiology seem easy compared to observing the pain of strangers. But I'm stubborn. I do not run. I will go back the next day. And the day after that.

My belly doesn't fit easily under the desk. I've made it through graduation, and this is the next hurdle: nursing boards. A Rite of passage. the *registered* in RN. My hands feel shaky, partly a result of my sitting for the exam, partly a result of the terbutaline I'm taking to prevent preterm labor. The amber bottle of pills sits on the corner of my desk. After hesitantly allowing me to leave the house at all, my midwife gave me specific instructions for self-dosing as needed to prevent contractions. She has forbidden stress in my life lest this impatient, growing child come too soon. Terbutaline effectively controls labor only if the patient's pulse is above one hundred, so it isn't so fabulous for stress reduction. Nonetheless, I hope it comes up as a test question.

Half of the test questions read like gibberish. Maybe Tolkien wrote the exam—in Elvish. My first degree was in liberal arts, but I never did love Tolkien. I should have finished *The Hobbit* after all. Who doesn't finish *The Hobbit?* This is some twist of karma. I will fail my boards, fail my baby, fail my life. I haven't studied much because of the ban on stress.

I remind myself that it won't matter, ten years from now, if I fail my boards the first time. The well-being of this child will matter. I take a deep breath, hunker down, and fill in the dots with my number two pencil. For two days I do this. During break, my former classmates and I congregate, somehow finding each other in the swarming mass of hopeful nursing school graduates: we the survivors of Wayne State University and Henry Ford Hospital. Most of us predict our own doom. "What did you say for the one on digoxin? I thought maybe it was all of the above, but I couldn't decide if it really caused purple hair to grow out your ears. It doesn't? No horns either? Damn."

Turns out I pass. My name badge says RN. The baby is fine. I have a license and a son. I'm still working on stress-free living.

The blinds are closed. The room is as dark as it can be in the midafternoon of a sunny Colorado day. The blue sky and sunshine are almost mocking, the atmosphere outside so incongruous with the atmosphere of the room.

Dappled sunlight reflects off the hospital bed frame. No one occupies the bed. The family is huddled in the corner: Mom, Dad, and their baby girl. The shoulders of the parents are hunched, heavy and laden, their eyes red and puffy. The mother cradles her first child, a baby she's had nine months of pregnancy to fall in love with. The cap on the baby's head hides the defect. She was born with anencephaly; her forebrain and cerebrum—the parts of her brain responsible for motor and sensory coordination and conscious thinking—did not develop. Most of her skull is missing. She has a rudimentary brain stem, the oldest part of the brain, the part responsible for breathing and reflexes. It's not enough to keep her alive for long. She will die within hours. Her face is peaceful; the rest of her tiny body is perfect.

This is my first newborn loss. It will not be my last. *It's not right that your birthday should also be your death day*, I think. I feel powerless. I'm filled with uncertainty, and I ask my charge nurse for suggestions. She shrugs a shoulder, not dismissively but resignedly. The answer is that there is no answer. I'll have to find my way. I don't know whether to leave them alone or stay with them. I feel like a blind man in an unfamiliar room, feeling my way through as best I can. It is, after all, not about me. I tell them to let me know what they need; it seems hollow. I check back periodically to let them know I'm available. Over the next couple hours, the baby's breathing becomes more labored. I tend to the mother's physical needs, making sure she's stable. She gave birth just a few hours ago. We talk about how the baby is doing. We talk about how beautiful she is. I protect their privacy at their request. They want their brief time as a family to themselves. The last time I see the baby before she dies, she nuzzles into her mother's breast, rooting, looking for food. It's a reflex in newborns, a key element of our survival as a species, one part of a primal relationship—the baby needs nourishment, and the mother needs to nourish. Tears well up in the mother's eyes again, and she tenderly strokes her baby's cheek. Dad leans across and kisses his daughter. I put a hand on each of their backs as my eyes well up, too. Is it OK for a nurse to cry with a patient? I again leave them alone with their grief. I don't want to intrude.

Not long afterward, the father nods to me from the doorway. He wipes his eyes with the back of his hand. When the doctor pronounces the baby's death, I go to take her. The doctor says they're ready, but I can't imagine that anyone could be ready to let go of a child. She's in her father's arms as he says good-bye to her. I hug her mother. We hold each other briefly, and we all cry. It's not a moment I'd have chosen, but it's a moment that has chosen me. I am present for a sacred moment—present physically and emotionally. It's the best I can do. It is neither heroic nor glamorous. I am a witness to overwhelming love and loss. I am, in some strange way, both honored and humbled.

I go home and hug my children. I squat down to their level, sitting on my heels as I often do. My bright, beautiful girl wraps her spindly arms around my neck, the tendrils of her hair tickling my nose. My toddling, smiling boy jumps on my back with the enthusiasm of a baseball player sliding into home plate. He wraps his arms around my neck. I am sandwiched between two miracles and overwhelmed with gratitude. I think they don't notice my tears. I hold them and want to never let go. They both plant wet, sticky, post-popsicle kisses on my cheeks. Cherry and grape. I love them so much it aches.

I need new kitchen chairs. The old ones have been beaten into submission by a kindergartner and a third grader. It's a simple enough task, and I have a few minutes before I have to pick the kids up from school. The shop is filled with refinished antique furniture, unaffordable on a nurse's wages, and unfinished new furniture that I can maybe manage. I'm greeted at the door by the fumes of wood stain and varnish. I browse for a few moments before I see him coming my way; Mr. Taylor has emerged from the back of the shop. My guilty hope was that he would not be in today, but I've been here before and I know the risk. He's elderly, lonely, and a talker. He asks what I'm looking for. I tell him, and he shows me some oak, mission-style antiques that I can nary afford. Then it starts.

"I got these on one of my last trips to the East Coast with my wife. Found 'em at an estate sale. They'd been in a barn for heaven only knows how long."

"Beautiful," I say as I sneak a furtive glance at my watch. The bell rings in ten minutes. It'll take me six minutes to get to the school. T minus four and counting.

"I don't travel anymore. It isn't the same without her. We had such fun on those trips. Auctions, estate sales . . . kept at it till the trailer was full, then came home. Our boys would man the store. Course they're busy with their own families now. Lucky to have grandkids, I am."

I've heard this story before, but I smile. "Sounds like a great life. Those grandkids are lucky to have you, too," I say. T minus three.

"The boys still help out, but the travel's not the same without my Millie. That's why I started carrying this unfinished furniture, ya see. Good quality but no travel. Just order it up from the catalog."

"I wish I'd met her," I say. T minus two.

"Say . . . you been in here before . . . haven't you? You're a nurse up there at the hospital, aren't you? My Millie was in that oncology ward in her last days. Those nurses were the best. Don't know what we woulda done without 'em."

Ah, the beauty and the curse of this small Colorado town. No anonymity. I smile and nod in response. T minus one.

"I was just up to the hospital myself," he tells me. "Didn't see you though . . ."

He wouldn't have. Although our town is relatively small, our hospital is not. It's a regional medical center. Also, I'm an Ob-gyn/nursery nurse. Unless he was pregnant, just had a baby, or weighed fewer than ten pounds himself, the odds of his seeing me were slim.

"Problems with my ticker," he continued.

That explains it—not pregnant. T minus zero. I've got to extricate myself from this conversation before my kids' school calls Social Services to report child abandonment.

"I'm sorry to hear that. You look well," I say. "Thanks for your help today," I add quickly before he has a chance to start in again. "I'll have to come back another time. I have to go get my kids."

"You go right on ahead. See you another time then!"

I head out the door. "Wait! Just one more thing!" I've started my exit too late already. I'm officially late. "I want you to know that nurses are God's angels on Earth. You remember that," he says.

"I will. Thank you for saying so. You take care, Mr. Taylor." I say.

I do a mental eye roll and scoff at his idealism as I rush to the car. An angel I am not. What I am is a busy working mother who has too many balls in the air and doesn't juggle especially well. Sometimes I feel as if I'm juggling swords. Or torches. Maybe flaming swords. At home, I sometimes yell at my kids, and I get impatient with my patients at work. Maybe my halo was knocked from my head by the flaming swords. It's more of an ankle bracelet, really. I'm sure it will look lovely with my support hose and the orthopedic nurses' shoes that are surely in my future. Anyway, a halo at work would only get in the way. The constant polishing to prevent tarnishing, the adjusting to make the tilt just so, the grabbing to prevent it from inadvertently falling on a baby. And the wings? I can't even imagine the maintenance. I don't spend more than five minutes on my hair. Who has time for wings?

But this is the life I have chosen. My work is meaningful, and it gives me time for my kids. I find them playing on the school playground, nonplussed. Turns out they are less affected than their mother by their temporary abandonment.

Mr. Taylor dies before I get back to his shop. I will miss him. I hope he had a good nurse in his last days.

Nurses have a longstanding tradition of eating their young. It starts in nursing school with a handful of militant nursing instructors. After school is over, it continues in the workplace.

Betty has been a nurse forever. Since before electricity, I'm pretty sure. She probably keeps leeches in her pocket for bloodletting. It could be my blood next.

"There are no washcloths in this bassinet drawer," she says.

"Sorry—I didn't get to it," I say.

"Someone's got to do it," she tells me. I feel like an errant schoolgirl, though I'm a few years out of school.

Phyllis, another leech-toting, Dark Ages nurse, comes around the corner. "Some of your patients don't have full water pitchers at their bedsides—do you know how important it is to them to have water?"

Seriously? I think, not foolish enough to say it. I've spent the last twelve hours multitasking: I took care of moms and babies, postop gynecological patients, and sick, pregnant women; I took vital signs, drew labs, read lab results, gave medications, admitted new patients, taught people how to care for their babies, helped with breastfeeding, discharged patients, put overwhelmed new mothers back together, monitored pregnant women and their unborn babies, talked to doctors (not all of whom qualify for congeniality awards, believe me), gave injections, hung IVs, answered call lights, and did paperwork—an endless, roiling sea of fucking paperwork. I ate a Snickers bar on the fly for lunch and haven't peed in eight hours. Last week, I saved a life. Two, actually. A pregnant woman was having a placental abruption—her placenta was pulling away from the wall of her uterus, depriving her baby of oxygen and causing her to bleed, potentially to death. I caught it, and a C-section was performed in time to save them both. What about that? Doesn't that count for anything? Washcloths and water pitchers? Who the hell cares? What I say aloud is, "It was really, really busy. I didn't even eat lunch."

"When is it *not* really busy?" asks Phyllis. "And how much good are you if you haven't eaten?"

Cannibalism is ugly, I think. I want to cry, but I don't.

On my drive home, after I've felt sorry for myself and licked my wounds (quite possibly induced by the leeches), I realize that they're right. It's nearly always busy and almost never about being a hero. It's about the mundane, the day to day. People need water and washcloths. It's work. Someone's got to do it, and leaving it for the next nurse is bad manners. I'm the only one who's likely to feel sorry that I haven't taken care of myself. Nurses need to eat and pee. This is a tough crowd. I am learning accountability: to my patients, to myself, and to my fellow nurses.

Betty and Phyllis become not only my mentors but my friends. I grow to love them, leeches and all.

I wear many hats at work, and I'm able to fill several roles in our women's and children's department. I'm flexible and don't mind it; it keeps things interesting. Today, I'm the transitional-care nurse. I'm catching babies. After they are born, they are my responsibility while they transition to life outside the womb. Most do well. The miracle happens without much intervention from me, but even after years of experience, I continue to feel apprehensive at the moment of delivery. Childbirth is messy and full of blood, other bodily fluids, and interesting odors. Babies all look lousy at delivery. Varying shades of blue are the most typical. Many are feisty and holler immediately, announcing their arrival with gusto. They pop their little lungs open and turn pink. Others enter the world and take a moment. They're in no hurry to breathe. Sometimes they need a little help, a reminder, maybe a little oxygen. Some need a lot of help. I've rushed more than one to the neonatal intensive care unit in my career. Most of the time, though, it's routine. I keep a close eye on vital signs for the first couple of hours; being born is a lot of work, and they could still turn on me. I give them routine newborn medications, help them eat, bathe them, and answer their parents' questions. Sometimes, lots of questions.

Today, I'm outnumbered six to one. Six babies in two hours and one baby nurse: me. My feet hurt from running between rooms and my back aches from leaning over babies. My hair feels like it might ignite momentarily from the heat of the radiant warmers, which help newborns to regulate their body temperatures but don't do a thing for menopausal nurses. I'm glad I don't use hairspray since an accelerant would surely cause combustion. That would be a lot of additional paperwork. I'm sure of it.

"You have such a happy job! You're so lucky!" says the grandmother of the baby born not more than ten minutes ago. I force my face into a smile, hoping it doesn't look like a grimace. This is not the first time I've heard this or something similar. I have, in fact, heard it ad nauseum for years. It makes me irritable. What she means, and I know this because I'm a mind reader, is that we do nothing but sit around all day, cuddling babies. She has no idea. The days of babies lined up in the nursery with a matronly nurse to watch over them are gone. They were gone before I started in this business, and I've been at it a while.

Don't misunderstand—it is happy most of the time. I love nothing more than to see first-time parents fall in love with their babies, the lights in their eyes when they come to love someone more than they ever thought possible. But we see it all. I've seen babies taken from their mothers by Social Services before they left the hospital; I've seen babies that maybe should have been taken. I've seen armed guards who kept watch over mothers who would return to jail. I've seen babies born as the result of rape and incest. I've seen babies withdraw from drugs because their mothers were addicts. And teen moms. Lots and lots of teen moms. I've held more than one crying baby while thinking, *Yeah, I'd cry, too, if I was going home with them.* I would try to banish the thought. I would try not to judge. Sometimes I did, but it wasn't my place.

The redeeming thing, the thing that gives me hope, is the love they all feel for their babies. Every one of them. They are occasionally incapable of caring for their children, but they love them nonetheless. It's both redeeming and tragic. Loving them is not always enough. If it were, it would be easy. Instead, it's messy. Life starts that way and continues that way. It doesn't proceed according to an obvious or understandable trajectory. It is messy and unpredictable, miraculous and wondrous. I am lucky. It's not always a happy job, but I am lucky.

Every day I go to work, I don my communication badge. It is not, as the name might suggest, something I earned in Girl Scouts after learning to speak in complex sentences with polysyllabic words. It's a little black device, about the size of a book of matches, that hangs from a lanyard around my neck. I can speak to my coworkers through this magic black box, which functions like a hands-free cell phone, only less reliably. It's better than nothing, especially after our move from an eighteen-bed floor to a shiny new one with thirty-two beds. When I started this job, we averaged a hundred births a month. That number has now doubled. Our new floor is a hundred yards long. A linoleum football field. We needed the space, and we need our little black boxes to communicate within it. I am the charge nurse on nearly every day I work. The role isn't new for me, but it has morphed into a job that is more managerial and less focused on patient care. Life in our new digs is a bit more complicated owing to the increased size and volume. It has become a sort of amalgamation of air traffic control, firefighting, and cat herding, with a den mother who doubles as a drill sergeant thrown in. I have a love-hate relationship with being the charge nurse. I also have a love-hate relationship with the little black box.

"Can you take a call from Sally Euler?" it asks me.

"Yes," I say.

"I'm sorry. I don't understand," says the black box.

"Yeess," I say. It is not sorry.

Sally asks which room I'd like to give to the next incoming patient and which nurse I'd like to give her to. We have only one room available, at the moment, so that's an easy decision. Jill will be her nurse. Jill will not be happy about it. She's already too busy.

"Call Jill Parker," I tell the box. I need to tell her she'll be getting a new patient.

"Did you say 'Michael Rodriguez'?" the box asks.

Michael Rodriquez? Wha? Not even close. "No," I say.

"OK. Let's try again," it says. The box cares not at all about my consternation.

Eventually, through the miracle of technology, I speak to Jill. She is, indeed, not happy, but I'm growing used to it. Someone is usually unhappy with me these days. It's the curse of the charge nurse. Some days I care, some I don't. At any rate, it gives me a chance to work on my people-pleasing and codependency issues. (If you ever meet a nurse who says she doesn't have people-pleasing and codependency issues, she's lying.)

"Can you talk to Marlene Nelson?" asks the box.

"Yes."

"Hey, Lori—where's the Doppler? I can't find it."

I don't know where it is, and I suspect she could find it as easily as I can, but I look anyway.

"Can you talk to Vicki Bridger?" The box again.

"Yes."

"Hi, Lori. It's Vicki." I know. The box keeps me well informed. "If anyone gets to leave early today, I'd like to. Just so you know."

Good Lord, it's not even eight o'clock. We still have eleven hours of this shift left. Go home early—yeah, right. Not happening in *this* lifetime. The grumbling in my head is loud.

"Can you talk to Gwen Chandler?" The box is relentless.

"Yeah, OK!" I say.

"I'm sorry. I don't understand," says the box. No shades of gray. Yes or no. The box will not have it any other way. It's good that the lanyard from which the godforsaken black box hangs has a breakaway clasp, or I might hang myself from it.

I am already irritable when one of my young charges walks into the nurses' station where I stand arguing with the box. Her hair hangs to the middle of her back. She has a pierced nose and tongue. Back in the day, we all pulled our hair back if it was longer than shoulder length. Jewelry was not allowed. Oh God, did I really just think, *back in the day?* I did. Damn. My young colleague reports to me that she's done something, well, stupid. Not life threateningly so but potentially harmful. When I confront her about her judgment and explain to her why I would have made a different decision, she replies with several justifications for her actions, none of which makes a bit of sense. I try another approach, telling her that I did not learn what I know about this particular situation in nursing school. I learned it from twenty years of nursing. I learned it from other nurses. We all learn from each other, and none of us knows everything. No harm came of her mistake, making this is a great learning opportunity.

Then I see it. The look. I know this look. It's the same one my daughter got when she became a teenager. The look that coincided, by her estimation, with the drop of my IQ into the single digits. The look that coincided, by my estimation, with the Pod People's replacement of my real daughter with someone who only looked like her. *That* look. I make a mental note to talk to hospital security about letting the Pod People in. The look is certainly not one of contrition, or humility, or receptiveness. It scares me. I want to send this young nurse to her room. Instead, I send her back to her patient's room to fix her mistake. I tell her to put her hair back and lose the jewelry while she's at it.

I sometimes fear that I've become that old, cranky, curmudgeonly nurse. I remember glass IV bottles and starched white uniforms. It makes me feel old and slightly weary. Some days, I have a hard time recalling how I felt when I was a beginner in this profession. I can recall the memories cognitively, but recalling them emotionally is more difficult. Some of the young nurses are overconfident, some overwhelmed. I relate more to the overwhelmed, but I get impatient and short-tempered even with them. At least I'm not a yeller, and I hope I'm not belittling. When I lament my lack of patience and my irascibility, I remember that I was raised by the likes of Betty and Phyllis, which is a little like being raised by wolves. I'm grateful to those women, and I turned out OK.

Some people say nursing is a calling. I never saw a burning bush or heard God's booming voice from on high. If I had, I might have attributed it to my recreational activities with pharmaceuticals back when I was getting my first degree in arts and humanities, which I suppose ultimately led me to nursing school. While I don't regret having gotten a degree that prepared me to be an aesthetic, well-read, and critically thinking human, job offers, other than those that involved phrases like *Do you want fries with that?* were not forthcoming. I had a baby girl, and I needed a way to make a reasonable living. That, and I wanted to save the world. Nursing seemed to be as good a way as any.

I had a nursing professor who used to espouse her disdain for the hearts that adorned nursing paraphernalia. The bags that said things like "Nurses have ♥," or the T-shirts that said "I ♥ a nurse." She said we needed to get rid of the damn hearts and put brains in their places. "We are not handmaidens for doctors or just pillow fluffers for patients." Her point was well-taken. In the beginning I resented that nursing was so stereotypically female. Touchy-feely, warm and fuzzy, suffocating in its wholesomeness. And I landed in Ob-gyn; it doesn't get much more touchy-feely than that. But each time I've ventured too far from that sphere, it has sucked me back in. I've surrendered. It seems to be where I belong, where I'm supposed to be. I have learned to celebrate that my profession is a nurturing one, to celebrate what I both bring and take from it as a nurse, a woman, a mother, a professional. I bring my brain and my heart. I've become a nurse almost in spite of myself. It's been a process, a journey. It has become part of who I am, whether I like it or not. Most days, I like it.

As it turns out, I haven't saved the world. I've had a hand in saving some lives and have, I hope, made small differences in the lives of many. Occasionally, patients express their gratitude. Some send us cards, some leave us chocolate. But external validation, the adoration and accolades of others, can't sufficiently make my job feel worth it. My job is worth it because I go home, on most days, with the feeling that I've at least broken even—I've put back at least as much as I've withdrawn from the karmic bank. It's a blessing in my life that I've been given the opportunity to be useful in my corner of the world. Today, that's enough for me.

LORI MULVIHILL *lives, writes, and works as an RN in Colorado, whose Rocky Mountains and blue skies she enjoys with her husband and their pack of dogs. She has raised two wonderfully human, creative children and is now pursuing her writing as they pursue adulthood.*